WORKBOOK FOR DIAGNOSTIC MEDICAL SONOGRAPHY

A Guide to Clinical Practice, Abdomen and Superficial Structures

WORKBOOK FOR DIAGNOSTIC MEDICAL SONOGRAPHY

A Guide to Clinical Practice, Abdomen and Superficial Structures

FOURTH EDITION

Diane M. Kawamura, PhD, RT(R), RDMS, FSDMS, FAIUM
Brady Presidential Distinguished Professor
Department of Radiologic Sciences
Weber State University
Ogden, Utah

Tanya D. Nolan, EdD, RT(R), RDMS
Associate Professor
Department of Radiologic Sciences
Weber State University
Ogden, Utah

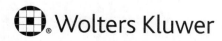. Wolters Kluwer

Philadelphia • Baltimore • New York • London
Buenos Aires • Hong Kong • Sydney • Tokyo

Senior Acquisitions Editor: Sharon R. Zinner
Development Editor: Amy Millholen
Editorial Coordinator: John Larkin
Marketing Manager: Shauna Kelley
Project Manager: Heidi Grauel
Production Project Manager: Linda Van Pelt
Design Coordinator: Joan Wendt
Manufacturing Coordinator: Margie Orzech
Prepress Vendor: S4Carlisle Publishing Services

Fourth edition

9 8 7 6 5

Printed in the United States

Library of Congress Cataloging-in-Publication Data

ISBN-13: 978-1-4963-8057-9
ISBN-10: 1-4963-8057-6

Cataloging-in-Publication data available on request from the Publisher.

LWW.com

CONTENTS

PART FOUR | SPECIAL STUDY SONOGRAPHY

Introduction

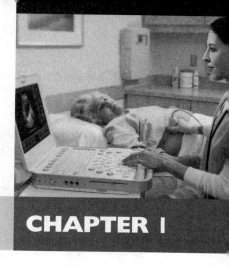

CHAPTER 1

REVIEW OF GLOSSARY TERMS

Matching

Match the terms with their definitions.

KEY TERMS

1. _____ anechoic

2. _____ echogenic

3. _____ echopenic

4. _____ isoechoic

5. _____ heterogeneous

6. _____ homogeneous

7. _____ hyperechoic

8. _____ hypoechoic

9. _____ specificity

10. _____ sensitivity

11. _____ accuracy

DEFINITIONS

a. Describes regions or portions on the sonogram where the echoes are not as bright as surrounding tissues or are less bright than normal

b. Defines how well an examination documents whatever disease or pathology is present

c. Describes tissues or organ structures on the sonogram having several different echo characteristics

d. Describes the sonographic appearance where the echoes are less echogenic or where a tissue or organ has few internal echoes

e. Describes a region or portion on the sonogram that appears echo-free

f. Defines the ability of the examination to find a disease that is present and not find a disease that is not present

g. Describes image echoes brighter than surrounding tissues or those brighter than what is normal for that tissue or organ

h. Describes where imaged echoes are of equal intensity

i. Describes structures of equal echo density

j. Defines how well an examination documents normal findings or excludes patients without disease

k. Describes an organ or tissue capable of producing echoes by reflecting the acoustic beam

ANATOMY AND PHYSIOLOGY REVIEW

Image Labeling

Complete the labels in the images that follow.

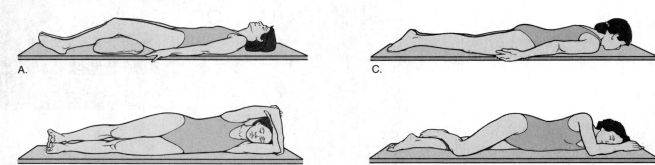

A.

C.

B.

D.

1. Patient positioning—What position is the patient in?

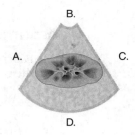

2. Longitudinal plane, left kidney

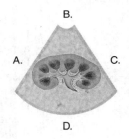

3. Coronal plane, left kidney

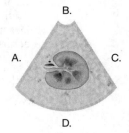

4. Transverse plane, left kidney

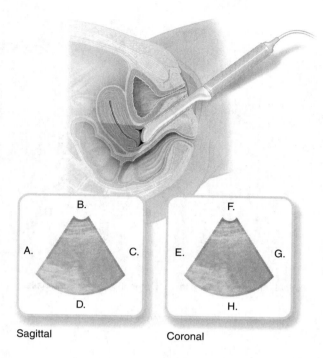

Sagittal   Coronal

5. Endovaginal planes

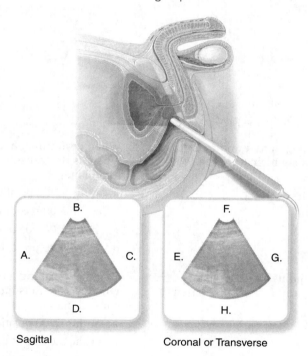

Sagittal   Coronal or Transverse

6. Endorectal planes

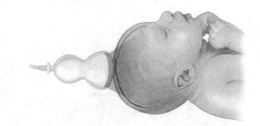

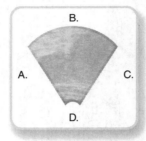 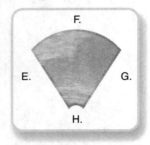

Sagittal: Anterior Fontanelle   Coronal: Anterior Fontanelle

7. Cranial fontanelle planes

CHAPTER REVIEW

Multiple Choice

Complete each question by circling the best answer.

1. When performing a neurosonography examination, the top of the image represents which scanning surface?
   a. anterior
   b. posterior
   c. superior
   d. inferior

2. When scanning in the longitudinal, sagittal plane, where is the transducer indicator located in relation to the organ of interest?
   a. at the 12:00 position
   b. at the 3:00 position
   c. at the 6:00 position
   d. at the 9:00 position

3. When scanning in the transverse plane, where is the transducer indicator located in relation to the organ of interest?
   a. at the 12:00 position
   b. at the 3:00 position
   c. at the 6:00 position
   d. at the 9:00 position

4. When performing a neonatal brain examination, where is the transducer indicator located in the sagittal plane?
   a. at the 12:00 position
   b. at the 3:00 position
   c. at the 6:00 position
   d. at the 9:00 position

5. When performing a neonatal brain examination, where is the transducer indicator located in the coronal plane?
   a. at the 12:00 position
   b. at the 3:00 position
   c. at the 6:00 position
   d. at the 9:00 position

6. When scanning in the longitudinal, sagittal plane, which of the following is NOT demonstrated in the image presentation?
   a. anterior
   b. cephalic
   c. right
   d. caudal

7. When scanning in the transverse plane on the anterior surface, which of the following is NOT demonstrated in the image presentation?
   a. posterior
   b. superior
   c. right
   d. left

8. Which of the following structures would NOT normally produce acoustic enhancement?
   a. urinary bladder
   b. simple kidney cyst
   c. gallbladder
   d. gallstone

9. Which of the following is NOT a sonographic criterion of a simple cyst?
   a. posterior acoustic shadowing
   b. anechoic center
   c. well-defined posterior wall
   d. edge-shadowing artifact

10. If a kidney stone is diagnosed with an abdominal sonogram but further testing reveals that the kidney is normal, what is this result called?
    a. a true-positive result
    b. a true-negative result
    c. a false-positive result
    d. a false-negative result

11. If a kidney stone is diagnosed with an abdominal sonogram and further testing also finds a kidney stone, what is this result called?
    a. a true-positive result
    b. a true-negative result
    c. a false-positive result
    d. a false-negative result

12. If the abdominal sonogram appears normal but a CT examination reveals a mass in the liver, what is this result called?
    a. a true-positive result
    b. a true-negative result
    c. a false-positive result
    d. a false-negative result

13. If the number of false-negative examinations increases, what happens to the sensitivity of the examination?
    a. The sensitivity will increase.
    b. False-negative results do not affect the sensitivity.
    c. The sensitivity will decrease.
    d. The sensitivity will remain the same.

14. What describes the likelihood of disease actually being present if the sonogram is positive?
    a. the negative predictive value
    b. the positive predictive value
    c. sensitivity
    d. specificity

15. Which term describes the ability of the examination to find diseases that are present and not find diseases that are not truly present?
    a. sensitivity
    b. specificity
    c. efficacy
    d. accuracy

Fill-in-the-Blank

1. The liver and spleen are located on opposite sides of the body and are therefore _____.

2. In directional terms, the lungs are _____ to the liver.

3. The _____ plane is a vertical plane that runs through the body and divides it into right and left sections.

4. The vertical plane that divides the body into equal right and left halves is called the _____ plane.

5. In the _____ position, the patient is lying supine on the examination table with his or her head lower than his or her feet.

6. The _____ plane is a horizontal plane that is perpendicular to the sagittal plane and divides the body into superior and inferior portions.

7. The _____ plane is a vertical plane that divides the body into anterior and posterior portions.

8. When performing an endovaginal examination in both the sagittal and coronal planes, the _____ anatomy is located at the apex of the image.

9. An organ may appear to have an abnormal echogenicity if disease is present or a poor examination technique is used, such as incorrect _____ settings.

10. Fluid-filled structures, such as the gallbladder, urinary bladder, or simple cysts, appear _____.

11. A normal testicle is described as _____, whereas a normal kidney appears _____.

12. The reduced echo amplitude found beyond a highly attenuating object such as a kidney stone is called an acoustic _____.

13. An artifact called _____ may be seen at the near wall of a simple cyst.

14. A _____ structure contains both solid and fluid components and will usually exhibit both anechoic and echogenic areas on the sonogram.

15. The preliminary report, which is also referred to as the _____ _____, should include the sonographic findings but should not include a diagnosis.

Short Answer

1. List the sonographic criteria that define a simple cyst.

2. What information should the sonographer include in his or her preliminary report? What information should be avoided?

3. What terminology can be used to describe a solid mass?

IMAGE EVALUATION/PATHOLOGY

Review the images and answer the following questions.

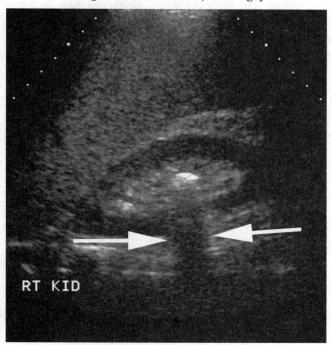

1. What is the name of the artifact that the large white arrows are pointing to?

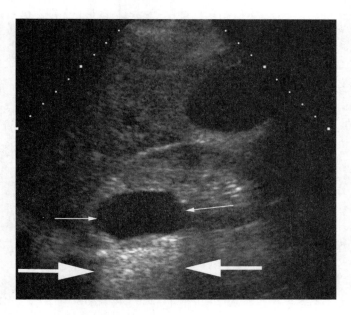

2. What type of artifact are the large white arrows pointing to? The small arrows are pointing to a cyst in the kidney. What term could be used to describe this structure?

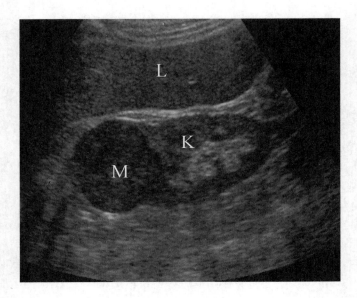

3. What term could you use to describe the echotexture of the kidney cortex (K) to the liver parenchyma (L)? What about the echotexture of the mass (M) to the kidney cortex? Would you describe the mass as heterogeneous or homogeneous?

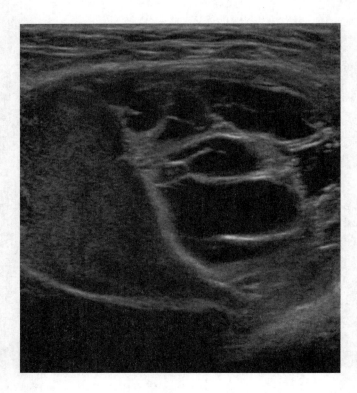

4. What one term would you use to describe the internal echo pattern of this mass?

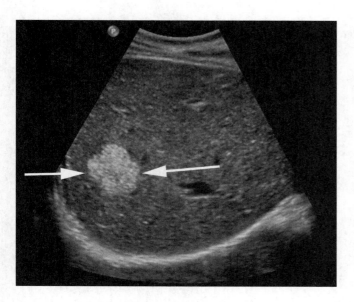

5. What term would be used to describe the echotexture of the mass (*arrows*) in comparison to the surrounding liver parenchyma?

CASE STUDY

1. A 38-year-old woman with right upper quadrant pain presents for an abdominal sonogram. What steps must the sonographer take prior to starting the examination that will enable him or her to provide the best possible examination?

2. You have been working on a research study. You have scanned 73 patients. Out of the 73 patients, 35 had a true-positive result and 31 had a true-negative result. There were 6 false-negative results and 1 false-positive result. From these statistics, calculate the sensitivity, specificity, and accuracy of the examination.

PART ONE

ABDOMINAL SONOGRAPHY

The Abdominal Wall and Diaphragm

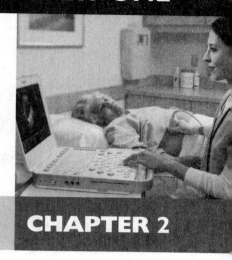

CHAPTER 2

REVIEW OF GLOSSARY TERMS

Matching

Match the key terms with their definitions.

KEY TERMS

1. _____ abscess

2. _____ ascites

3. _____ aponeurosis

4. _____ ecchymosis

5. _____ erythema

6. _____ fascia

7. _____ linea alba

8. _____ omphalocele

9. _____ peristalsis

10. _____ pleural effusion

11. _____ pneumothorax

12. _____ rectus abdominis

DEFINITIONS

a. Redness of the skin due to inflammation

b. Long, vertical, paired abdominal muscles that run from the xiphoid process to the symphysis pubis

c. Skin discoloration caused by the leakage of blood into the subcutaneous tissues

d. Cavity containing dead tissue and pus that forms due to an infectious process

e. Fibrous tissue network that is richly supplied by blood vessels and nerves located between the skin and the underlying structures

f. Accumulation of serous fluid in the peritoneal cavity

g. Rhythmic contraction of the GI tract that propels food through it

h. Fibrous structure that runs down the midline of the abdomen from the xiphoid process to the symphysis pubis

i. Fluid accumulation in the pleural cavity

j. Collapsed lung that occurs when air leaks into the space between the chest wall and lung

k. Layers of flat fibrous sheets composed of strong connective tissue, which serve as tendons to attach muscles to fixed points

l. Congenital defect in the midline abdominal wall that allows abdominal organs to protrude through the wall into the base of the umbilical cord

ANATOMY AND PHYSIOLOGY REVIEW

Image Labeling

Complete the labels in the images that follow.

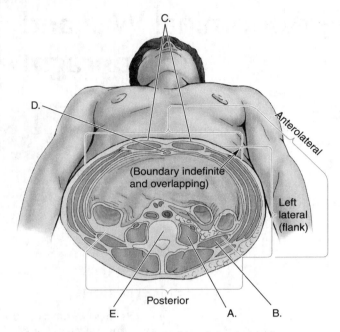

1. Transverse section of the abdominal wall

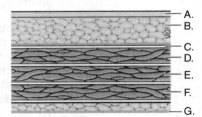

2. Subcutaneous layers of the abdominal wall

CHAPTER REVIEW

Multiple Choice

Complete each question by circling the best answer.

1. Which of the following has the primary function of attaching muscles to fixed points?
   a. superficial fascia
   b. deep fascia
   c. subcutaneous tissue
   d. aponeuroses

2. Which of the following muscles is not a paired muscle?
   a. pyramidalis muscle
   b. external oblique
   c. rectus abdominis
   d. transverse abdominis

3. Which of the following is an anatomical area, where vessels can enter and exit the abdominal cavity, and is a potential site for hernias?
   a. linea alba
   b. inguinal canal
   c. umbilicus
   d. rectus sheath

4. Which of the following is a true statement about the right crus of the diaphragm?
   a. It can be seen sonographically anterior to the abdominal aorta.
   b. It is shorter than the left crus of the diaphragm.

c. It can be seen anterior to the IVC.

d. It appears anterior to the caudate lobe.

5. Which of the following muscles is not part of the anterolateral abdominal wall?

   a. pyramidalis muscle

   b. psoas muscle

   c. rectus abdominis

   d. external oblique

6. Which statement regarding the diaphragm is FALSE?

   a. The right dome of the diaphragm is slightly higher than the left.

   b. The diaphragmatic apertures allow the esophagus, blood vessels, and nerves to pass between the chest and abdomen.

   c. The central portion of the diaphragm descends during inspiration and ascends during expiration.

   d. Due to diaphragmatic contraction, the IVC dilates during inspiration.

7. Which transducer is best suited for a sonographic examination of the superficial abdominal wall?

   a. 12 MHz linear array

   b. 4 MHz curved array

   c. 3 MHz phased array

   d. 4 MHz linear array

8. Which of the following is an inflammatory response?

   a. hematoma

   b. hernia

   c. abscess

   d. lipoma

9. In order to determine if an abscess is intraperitoneal or extraperitoneal, what structure must the sonographer demonstrate?

   a. linea alba

   b. peritoneal line

   c. rectus abdominus

   d. diaphragm

10. Which of the following may be a contraindication to sonography-guided aspiration?

   a. septations within the abscess

   b. particulate debris floating within the abscess

   c. an anechoic abscess with increased through transmission

   d. an echogenic abscess

11. Which of the following statements regarding hematomas is FALSE?

   a. Postsurgical hematomas are usually retroperitoneal.

   b. The echogenicity and sonographic appearance of a hematoma will vary depending on its age.

   c. The most common superficial abdominal wall hematomas occur within the rectus sheath.

   d. Hematomas are associated with muscular trauma that results in hemorrhage.

12. What is the most common content in an abdominal wall hernia?

   a. liver

   b. bowel

   c. free fluid

   d. fat

13. Which of the following is not a ventral hernia?

   a. umbilical

   b. inguinal

   c. hypogastric

   d. epigastric

14. What is the most common type of ventral hernia?

   a. umbilical

   b. inguinal

   c. hypogastric

   d. epigastric

15. Which of the following is the most common benign tumor of the abdominal wall?

   a. desmoid tumor

   b. sarcoma

   c. neuroma

   d. lipoma

16. Which of the following typically occurs when a nerve is damaged during surgery?

   a. desmoid tumor

   b. sarcoma

   c. neuroma

   d. lipoma

17. Which of the following is another term for pleural effusion?

   a. hydrothorax

   b. ascites

   c. eventration

   d. pneumothorax

18. Which of the following is an abnormal elevation of the diaphragm due to a developmental anomaly?
    a. pleural effusion
    b. eventration
    c. diaphragmatic paralysis
    d. diaphragmatic hernia

19. Over half of infants born with a congenital diaphragmatic hernia die from what medical condition?
    a. cardiac failure
    b. infection

    c. renal failure
    d. respiratory failure

20. Which of the following structures is usually not seen in the thoracic cavity in a fetus with a congenital diaphragmatic hernia?
    a. liver
    b. spleen
    c. stomach
    d. linea alba

Fill-in-the-Blank

1. The human body is divided into the ventral and dorsal cavities. The ventral cavity is separated by the diaphragm into the _____ cavity and the _____ cavity.

2. The superficial fascia inferior to the umbilicus is divided into two layers: the _____ fascia, a fatty layer containing small vessels and nerves, and the _____ fascia, which is a deep membranous layer.

3. The _____ _____ lines the abdominopelvic cavity and is formed by a single layer of epithelial cells and supporting connective tissue.

4. The _____ _____ is a fibrous compartment that contains the rectus abdominis, pyramidalis muscle, blood and lymphatic vessels, and nerves.

5. The posterior abdominal wall is composed of three paired muscles: the _____ _____, _____, and _____ _____.

6. When evaluating a superficial lesion in the abdominal wall, a _____ _____ may be used to eliminate the "main bang" artifact.

7. Sonographically, the diaphragm is seen as a thin _____ band in children and adults and as a _____ band in fetuses.

8. Three main categories of disease that affect the abdominal wall include _____, _____, and _____ changes.

9. The four clinical indications of an inflammatory response are _____, _____, _____, and _____.

10. The shape of an abscess can vary, but the typical shape is _____ or _____.

11. If edema is present after an injury, a contused abdominal muscle may appear _____ and more _____.

12. Superficial abdominal wall hematomas most commonly occur within the _____ _____.

13. Discoloration of the abdominal wall called _____ and a falling _____ value are often clinical signs of a rectus sheath hematoma.

14. A _____ is a collection of serum that results from a surgical procedure or from the liquefaction of a he-matoma and typically appears anechoic to hypoechoic sonographically.

15. The two main categories of abdominal wall hernias are _____ and _____.

16. Two complications that can occur with midline hernias include _____, which can compromise the blood supply and cause ischemia, and _____, which occurs when the contents of the sac cannot be pushed back into the abdominal cavity.

17. When evaluating a hernia with sonography, the _____ _____ can be used to demonstrate the widening of the hernia and movement of the hernia contents.

18. Sonographically, a _____ _____ is diagnosed when fluid is visualized superior to the diaphragm.

19. Paralysis of one hemidiaphragm can be detected sonographically by showing _____ or _____ motion on the affected side and normal or _____ motion on the contralateral side.

20. A diaphragmatic hernia allows _____ contents such as _____, _____, and _____ to enter the thoracic cavity.

Short Answer

1. Sonographically, how would one distinguish ascites from a pleural effusion?

2. Describe the process of abscess formation and resolution.

3. You receive a request to perform an examination of the anterior abdominal wall on a patient with a recent history of abdominal surgery. The area surrounding the incision is red and warm to touch, and the referring physician is concerned about the presence of an abscess. What techniques and precautions will you use to limit the spread of infection to this and subsequent patients?

4. A 68-year-old man presents with a clinical history of an umbilical hernia post aortic aneurysm repair. You scan over the area and are not sure that you can visualize the hernia. What technique will you use to hopefully make the hernia more visible, and what five things you must evaluate when performing an examination on an abdominal hernia?

5. You receive a request to perform a portable chest sonogram in the ICU on a patient with suspected right hemidia-phragmatic paralysis. Describe the exam protocol you will follow and what factors you will be looking for.

IMAGE EVALUATION/PATHOLOGY

Review the images and answer the following questions.

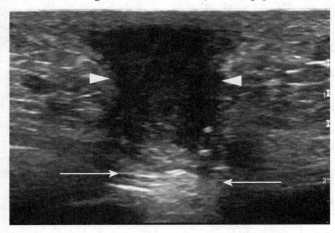

1. This image was taken at the level of the umbilicus and represents a periumbilical abscess (*arrowheads*). How would you describe the mass sonographically? What are the long arrows pointing to? Why does that occur?

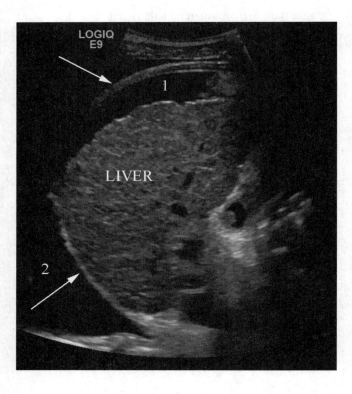

2. What anatomic structure are the arrows pointing to? What does the number *1* represent? What does the number *2* represent?

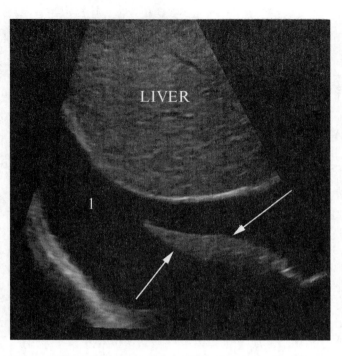

3. What anatomic structure are the arrows pointing to? What does the number *1* represent?

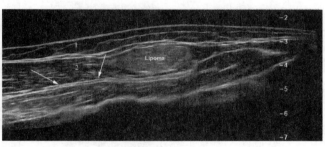

4. Describe the sonographic appearance of the lipoma seen within the anterior abdominal wall. What layer does the number *1* represent? Number *2*? What structure do the arrows represent?

CASE STUDY

Review the images and answer the following questions.

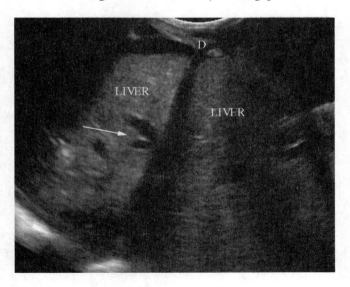

1. A neonate presents for an abdominal sonogram a few hours after delivery to follow up an abnormality seen on a prenatal sonogram. This image was taken in the right upper quadrant and demonstrates the diaphragm indicated by the letter *D*. Liver is seen both superior and inferior to the diaphragm. What is the likely diagnosis? What causes this abnormality, and what is the most common complication associated with it?

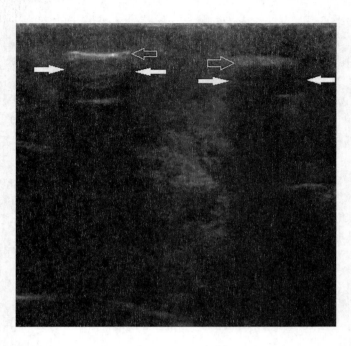

2. A patient presents for an abdominal wall sonography examination with a recent history of a laparoscopic colon operation. The patient now presents with pain, tenderness, and erythema around the laparoscopic incision site. Describe the sonographic appearance and discuss the probable diagnosis based on the history and image. What is the likely treatment for this patient?

The Peritoneal Cavity

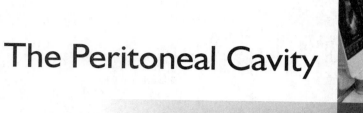

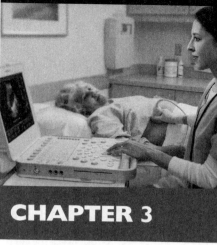

CHAPTER 3

REVIEW OF GLOSSARY TERMS

Matching

Match the key terms with their definitions.

KEY TERMS

1. _____ abscess
2. _____ ascites
3. _____ bare area
4. _____ biloma
5. _____ FAST scan
6. _____ hematoma
7. _____ hemoperitoneum
8. _____ hilum
9. _____ iatrogenic
10. _____ lymphocele
11. _____ mesentery
12. _____ peritoneal organs
13. _____ parietal peritoneum
14. _____ retroperitoneal organs
15. _____ seroma
16. _____ visceral peritoneum

DEFINITIONS

a. Caused by treatment; either intentional or unintentional
b. Fluid collection composed of blood products located adjacent to or surrounding transplanted organs
c. Surface area of a peritoneal organ devoid of peritoneum
d. Peritoneum encasing peritoneal organs
e. Pocket of infection typically containing pus, blood, and degenerating tissue
f. Solid organs within the peritoneal cavity that are covered by visceral peritoneum
g. Collection of bile that can occur with trauma or rupture of the biliary tract
h. Area of an organ where blood vessels, lymph, and nerves enter and exit
i. Free fluid within the peritoneal cavity
j. An extravasated collection of lymph
k. Peritoneum lining the walls of the peritoneal cavity
l. Two layers of fused peritoneum that conduct nerves, lymph, and blood vessels between the small bowel/colon and the posterior peritoneal cavity wall
m. Triage ultrasound examination performed to detect free fluid that would indicate bleeding
n. Organs posterior to the parietal peritoneum, which are typically covered on their anterior surface or fatty capsule by parietal peritoneum
o. Extravasated collection of blood within the peritoneal cavity
p. Extravasated collection of blood localized within a potential space or tissue

ANATOMY AND PHYSIOLOGY REVIEW

Image Labeling

Complete the labels in the images that follow.

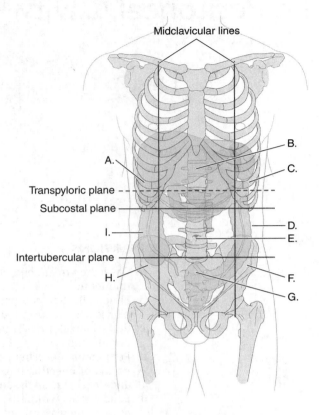

1. Addison lines—Label the nine abdominopelvic regions.

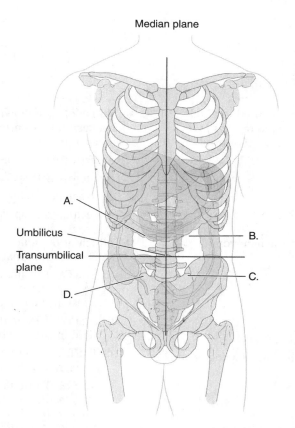

Median plane

A.

Umbilicus

B.

Transumbilical plane

C.

D.

2. Quadrants of the abdominopelvic cavity—Label the four quadrants.

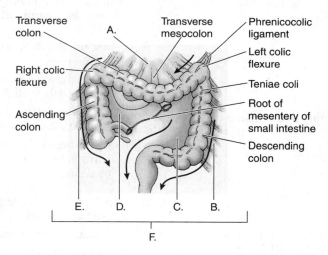

Transverse colon

A.

Transverse mesocolon

Phrenicocolic ligament

Right colic flexure

Left colic flexure

Teniae coli

Ascending colon

Root of mesentery of small intestine

Descending colon

E.   D.   C.   B.

F.

3. Potential spaces—Label the potential spaces.

CHAPTER REVIEW

Multiple Choice

Complete each question by circling the best answer.

1. Which of the following methods is used to divide the abdominopelvic cavity into nine regions by drawing two vertical and two horizontal lines?
   a. McBurney lines
   b. Murphy lines
   c. xyphoid lines
   d. Addison lines

2. What term refers to peritoneum that surrounds the abdominal organs?
   a. visceral peritoneum
   b. hilar peritoneum
   c. parietal peritoneum
   d. retroperitoneum

3. The lesser sac contains which of the following organs?
   a. liver
   b. stomach
   c. pancreas
   d. The lesser sac does not contain any organs.

4. Which of the following spaces is most likely to contain a pancreatic pseudocyst?
   a. lesser sac
   b. greater sac
   c. hepatorenal space
   d. left paracolic gutter

5. Which of the following is not another name for the rectouterine space?
   a. pouch of Douglas
   b. posterior cul-de-sac
   c. rectovaginal pouch
   d. prevesicle space

6. Which of the following potential spaces is commonly referred to as Morrison pouch?
   a. the left anterior subphrenic space
   b. the left posterior suprahepatic space
   c. the hepatorenal space
   d. the right subphrenic space

7. Which of the following potential spaces is located between the anterior wall of the urinary bladder and the pubic symphysis?
   a. vesicorectal space
   b. uterovesicle space
   c. space of Retzius
   d. rectouterine space

8. Which of the following potential spaces is located between the posterior urinary bladder and the anterior uterus?
   a. vesicorectal space
   b. uterovesicle space
   c. space of Retzius
   d. rectouterine space

9. Which of the following statements regarding the FAST scan examination is FALSE?
   a. The FAST examination is very effective in diagnosing causes of acute abdominal pain such as gallstones and kidney stones.
   b. The FAST examination is used to search for free fluid in cases of blunt abdominal trauma.
   c. FAST is an acronym for Focused Assessment with Sonography in Trauma.
   d. The FAST examination has proven to be sensitive in detecting as little as 200 mL of free fluid within the peritoneal cavity and 20 mL of fluid within the pleural cavity.

10. Which of the following statements regarding a sonographic examination of peritoneal cavity is FALSE?
   a. Ascites will demonstrate bowel moving freely within it.
   b. Cystic masses typically have sharp corners and angles as they fill the potential spaces.
   c. Changing patient position can be used to demonstrate the movement of free fluid.
   d. Cystic masses may demonstrate a mass-effect on surrounding tissues and tend to have a round or oval shape.

11. Which of the following is typically associated with transudative ascites?
   a. inflammatory bowel disease
   b. ovarian cancer
   c. congestive heart failure
   d. peritonitis

12. Ascites does not typically collect in which of the following potential spaces?
   a. Morrison pouch
   b. pouch of Douglas
   c. paracolic gutters
   d. pleural space

13. Due to the high frequency of appendicitis and duo-denal ulcers, what is the most common potential space for a peritoneal abscess?

   a. right subphrenic space

   b. hepatorenal space

   c. left anterior subphrenic space

   d. space of Retzius

14. Which of the following statements regarding a peritoneal abscess is FALSE?

   a. The abscess may appear as a thick-walled fluid collection with internal debris.

   b. Color Doppler will frequently demonstrate internal vascularity.

   c. An abscess may be located in a potential space or next to an inflamed or perforated organ.

   d. A peritoneal abscess may be the result of a surgical complication.

15. A large hematoma may be associated with a decrease in which laboratory value?

   a. amylase

   b. white blood count

   c. bilirubin

   d. hematocrit

16. What is the common sonographic appearance of a lymphocele?

   a. hypoechoic collection with thick septations

   b. simple anechoic collection with possible thin septations

   c. complex mass with calcifications

   d. thick-walled collection with internal septations

17. What term describes an interventional procedure performed to remove ascites from the peritoneal cavity?

   a. thoracentesis

   b. fine-needle aspiration

   c. percutaneous abscess drainage

   d. paracentesis

18. Which fluid collection contains urine and is associated with a rupture of the urinary tract?

   a. biloma

   b. urinoma

   c. seroma

   d. lymphocele

19. Which of the following statements regarding omental caking is FALSE?

   a. Omental caking is a thickening of the greater omentum from malignant infiltration.

   b. Nodular masses may be seen sonographically deep to the anterior wall.

   c. Simple transudative ascites is frequently associated with omental caking.

   d. Omental caking is commonly associated with cancers of the ovary, stomach, and colon.

20. Which of the following organs is NOT located within the peritoneal cavity?

   a. liver

   b. pancreas

   c. spleen

   d. gallbladder

Fill-in-the-Blank

1. Addison lines divide the abdomen into nine regions. Those regions are the right and left _____, right and left _____, right and left _____, and the central regions _____, _____, and _____.

2. The abdominopelvic cavity is also frequently divided into four quadrants. Those quadrants are the _____, _____, _____, and _____.

3. The largest body cavity is called the _____ _____, which encompasses the abdomen and pelvis.

4. The thin sheet of tissues that divides the abdominal cavity into the peritoneal and retroperitoneal compartments is called the _____ _____.

5. The lesser sac lies immediately posterior to the _____.

6. The greater omentum divides the greater sac into two compartments: the _____ _____, which means above the colon, and the _____ _____, which means below the colon.

7. The right and left _____ _____ are potential spaces along the lateral borders of the peritoneal cavity that allows fluids to travel between the supracolic and infracolic compartments.

8. When a patient is supine, the most gravity-dependent portion of the abdominal cavity is the _____ _____. This potential space should always be checked for free fluid during the sonographic examination.

9. When a female patient is in the supine position, the _____ _____ is the most gravity-dependent portion of the pelvic cavity.

10. When a male patient is in the supine position, the _____ _____ is the most gravity-dependent portion of the pelvic cavity.

11. _____ ascites typically has a simple appearance because it is characterized by a lack of protein and cellular material.

12. _____ ascites has a more complex and echogenic appearance because fluid seeps out from blood vessels and contains a large amount of protein and cellular material.

13. The presence of _____ within an abscess may cause a "dirty" posterior shadow.

14. Free blood within the peritoneal cavity is called _____; once the blood organizes into a focal area or clot, the collection is called a _____.

15. _____ _____ results when a benign appendiceal or ovarian adenoma ruptures, spilling epithelial cells into the peritoneum, causing _____ _____ to accumulate within the peritoneal cavity.

16. Seromas typically occur _____ in the postsurgical period, whereas _____ are typically slower to develop and may present 4 to 8 weeks after surgery, helping to establish a more definitive diagnosis between the two similar-appearing fluid collections.

17. Mesenteric cysts may occur anywhere along the mesentery but are most commonly found originating from the _____ _____ mesentery.

18. The term _____ describes the enlargement of lymph nodes that can result from _____ diseases such as colitis or malignancies such as lymphoma or colon cancer.

19. Peritoneal mesothelioma is a rare malignant tumor of the peritoneum that is associated with exposure to _____.

20. A paracentesis may be done for _____ purposes to remove a small amount of fluid for laboratory testing or for _____ purposes to relieve pain and pressure that the patient may be experiencing due to a large volume of ascites.

Short Answer

1. What purpose does the greater omentum serve?

2. Explain the protocol used during a FAST examination. When and where is this procedure performed?

3. What are three common causes of ascites? Where is ascites most likely to accumulate?

4. Describe the sonographic appearance of a peritoneal abscess. Where might an abscess be located?

5. What is the purpose of the peritoneal membrane?

IMAGE EVALUATION/PATHOLOGY

Review the images and answer the following questions.

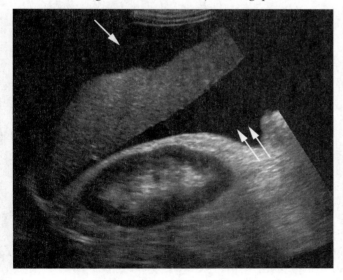

1. Which potential space is the *single arrow* pointing to? Which potential space is the *double arrow* pointing to? What pathology is seen in this image?

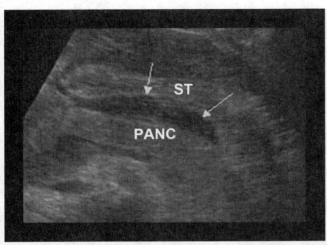

2. What potential space are the *arrows* pointing to? What pathologies might collect here?

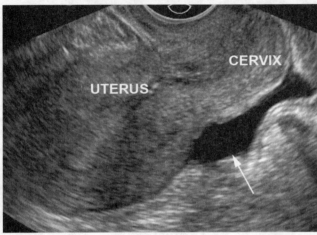

3. What potential space is the *arrow* pointing to? Why is this space significant?

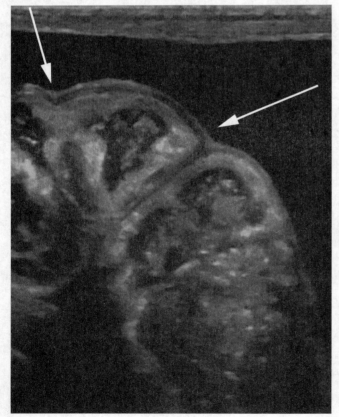

4. What type of ascites is seen in this image? What pathologies could have resulted in this type of ascites? What structure are the *arrows* pointing to?

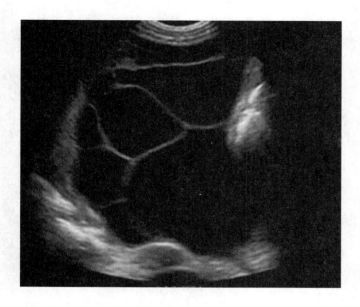

5. What type of ascites is seen in this image? How would you describe the ascites? What pathologies could have resulted in this type of ascites?

CASE STUDY

Review the image and answer the following questions.

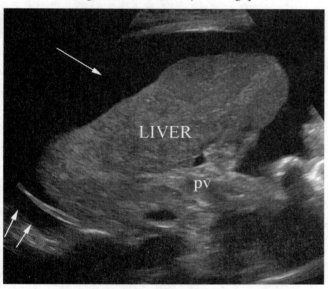

1. A 62-year-old man with a history of liver disease presents for an abdominal sonogram with a history of abdominal distention and pain. Your examination reveals an echogenic, irregular shrunken liver consistent with cirrhosis. You also discover portal vein thrombosis (*PV*) as the portal vein is filled with echogenic material and no color flow is identified. What pathology is the *arrow* pointing to? What is the *double arrow* pointing to? What procedure could be done to relieve the patient's symptoms of abdominal distention?

Vascular Structures

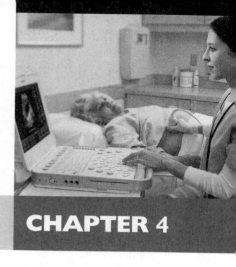

CHAPTER 4

REVIEW OF GLOSSARY TERMS

Matching

Match the key terms with their definitions.

KEY TERMS

1. _____ anastomosis

2. _____ aneurysm

3. _____ arteriovenous fistula

4. _____ ectasia

5. _____ endograft

6. _____ graft

7. _____ prosthesis

8. _____ pseudoaneurysm

9. _____ thrombosis

DEFINITIONS

a. Any tissue or organ for implantation or transplantation

b. Dilatation, expansion, or distention

c. Connection between two vessels

d. Focal dilatation of an artery caused by a structural weakness in the wall

e. An artificial substitute for a body part

f. A metallic stent covered with fabric and placed inside an aneurysm to prevent rupture

g. The formation of a clot in a blood vessel

h. Connection allowing communication between an artery and vein

i. Caused by a hematoma that forms as a result of a leaking hole in an artery

ANATOMY AND PHYSIOLOGY REVIEW

Image Labeling

Complete the labels in the images that follow.

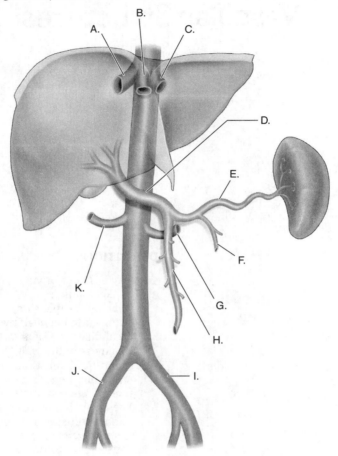

1. Abdominal vasculature

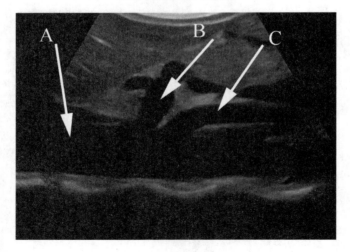

2. Abdominal vasculature

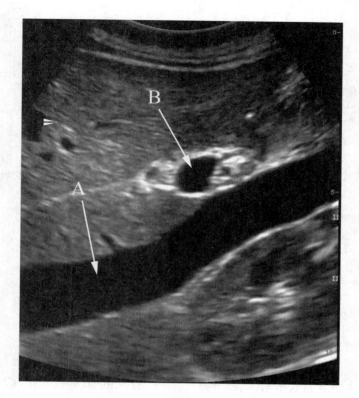

3. Abdominal vasculature

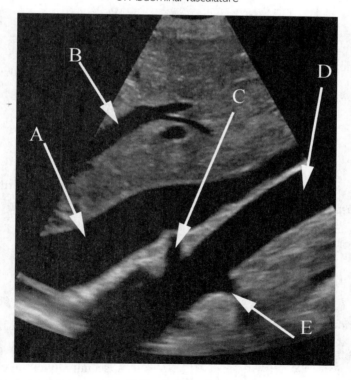

4. Abdominal vasculature

CHAPTER REVIEW

Multiple Choice

Complete each question by circling the best answer.

1. Which is the innermost layer of a vessel wall?
   a. tunica intima
   b. tunica media
   c. tunica adventitia
   d. tunica serosa

2. Which of the following statements regarding arteries and veins is FALSE?
   a. The walls of arteries and veins contain the same three layers.
   b. Both arteries and veins contain valves to keep blood moving.
   c. Because the walls of veins contain less muscle, they are more easily compressed.
   d. Arteries have a thicker muscle layer and therefore maintain a constant shape.

3. The compression of the left renal vein between the aorta and the SMA is referred to as the:
   a. sandwich effect
   b. Murphy phenomenon
   c. compartment syndrome
   d. nutcracker phenomenon

4. Which of the following veins does NOT drain into the IVC?
   a. portal vein
   b. middle hepatic vein
   c. left renal vein
   d. right renal vein

5. Which vessel courses posterior to the SMA and anterior to the aorta?
   a. superior mesenteric vein
   b. splenic vein
   c. left renal vein
   d. left gastric vein

6. Which vessel lies posterior to the bile duct and anterior to the portal vein?
   a. hepatic vein
   b. hepatic artery
   c. gastroduodenal artery
   d. celiac axis

7. Which vein is formed by the confluence of the superior mesenteric vein and the splenic vein?
   a. celiac axis
   b. portal vein

c. inferior vena cava
   d. main hepatic vein

8. Which of the following describes the location of the celiac axis to the origin of the superior mesenteric artery?
   a. cephalad
   b. caudal
   c. medial
   d. lateral

9. Which vessel lies posterior to the IVC?
   a. left renal vein
   b. right renal vein
   c. left renal artery
   d. right renal artery

10. The portal vein carries blood to the liver from the:
    a. aorta
    b. IVC
    c. splenic artery
    d. intestines

11. What is an aneurysm that is uniform in nature called?
    a. saccular
    b. fusiform
    c. dissecting
    d. congenital

12. How large must the aortic diameter be to diagnose an aortic aneurysm?
    a. 2 cm
    b. 3 cm
    c. 4 cm
    d. 5 cm

13. What is the typical sonographic appearance of an aortic dissection?
    a. a uniform dilation of the wall of the aorta
    b. a dilation of one side of the aorta, typically the left
    c. discontinuity of the wall of the aorta with a large hematoma surrounding the vessel
    d. thin linear flap seen pulsating within the aortic lumen with blood flow visible on both sides of the flap

14. At what size does risk of rupture greatly increase in an abdominal aortic aneurysm?
    a. 3 cm
    b. 5 cm

c. 7 cm

d. 9 cm

15. Which of the following is NOT a complication of aortic endografts?

a. endoleaks

b. abscess

c. dissecting aneurysm

d. pseudoaneurysm

16. What is the most common clinical symptom of renal artery stenosis?

a. abdominal pain

b. hypertension

c. increased urinary output

d. pulsatile abdominal mass

17. Mesenteric insufficiency results from a hemodynamically significant stenosis or occlusion of two out of three of the vessels that supply the intestinal tract. Which vessels are they?

a. portal vein, inferior mesenteric vein, superior mesenteric vein

b. portal artery, inferior mesenteric artery, hepatic artery

c. superior mesenteric artery, celiac axis, inferior mesenteric artery

d. gastroduodenal artery, hepatic artery, splenic artery

18. What happens when blood flow in the IVC is obstructed?

a. The entire IVC will become dilated.

b. The IVC will dilate proximal to the obstruction.

c. The IVC will dilate distal to the obstruction.

d. The IVC has thick walls and does not change in diameter.

19. What is the most common cause of IVC obstruction?

a. tumor due to renal cell carcinoma

b. thrombus from extension of DVT

c. right-sided heart failure

d. portal hypertension

20. Which of the following vessels must be evaluated to rule out "Budd–Chiari" disease?

a. aorta and celiac axis

b. renal veins and IVC

c. portal veins and hepatic veins

d. IVC and hepatic veins

21. What is the most likely cause of portal hypertension?

a. congestive heart failure

b. cirrhosis of the liver

c. dehydration

d. enlargement of the spleen

22. Which of the following is NOT characteristic of a vascular stenosis?

a. poststenotic dilatation of the vessel

b. vessel lumen visibly narrowed at the stenosis by calcified plaque

c. markedly decreased Doppler velocities at the level of the stenosis

d. poststenotic turbulence

23. Which type of aneurysm typically has a neck and demonstrates a swirling pattern on color Doppler?

a. dissecting

b. pseudoaneurysm

c. fusiform

d. mycotic

24. When a patient has an abdominal aortic aneurysm, what is the greatest concern?

a. the presence of thrombus

b. dissection

c. rupture

d. extension into the iliac arteries

25. Which of the following statements regarding portal hypertension is FALSE?

a. Portal hypertension is typically caused by increased hepatic vascular resistance.

b. The diameter of the portal vein is almost always decreased in cases of portal hypertension.

c. Portal hypertension can also be caused by Budd–Chiari syndrome.

d. Portal hypertension can result in collateral formation involving the coronary vein, gastroesophageal veins, and splenorenal veins.

Fill-in-the-Blank

1. Arteries and veins are composed of three layers: the _____ _____, _____
_____, and the _____ _____. The _____ _____ is thicker in
arteries and is largely responsible for their elasticity and contractility.

2. The aorta originates off of the _____ _____; once it penetrates the diaphragm, it is called the
_____ _____ and, finally, bifurcates into the right and left _____ _____
arteries.

3. The three branches of the celiac axis are the _____ _____, the _____
_____ _____, and the _____ _____.

4. The CA, SMA, and IMA originate from the _____ aspect of the aorta, whereas the right and left renal
arteries arise from the _____ aspect of the aorta.

5. The inferior vena cava is formed by the junction of the right and left _____ _____
_____, courses through the abdominal cavity, entering into the thoracic cavity to empty into the
_____ _____ of the heart.

6. The normal IVC will change caliber with respiratory maneuvers; _____ with inspiration due to the decreased
pressure within the thoracic cavity, _____ during expiration, and _____ with suspended respiration.
During the Valsalva maneuver, the IVC lumen _____.

7. The portal vein is formed by the junction of the _____ _____ and the _____
_____ _____ at the _____ _____, immediately posterior to the neck of
the pancreas.

8. _____ is a form of arteriosclerosis that is characterized by an accumulation of lipids, blood products,
and sometimes calcium deposits along the intimal lining of the arteries.

9. A _____ aneurysm is a protrusion toward one side or the other, unlike a fusiform aneurysm, which is
more uniform.

10. When an abdominal aortic aneurysm is diagnosed, the _____ arteries and _____ arteries
should also be examined to evaluate for extension of the aneurysm.

11. Aortic _____ is a separation of the layers of the aortic wall that typically presents with extreme chest or
abdominal pain.

12. Iliac artery aneurysms are most often a continuation of an _____ _____ _____
and tend to be _____.

13. EVAR stands for _____ _____ _____ _____.

14. A pulsatile anechoic mass at the anastomosis of an endograft that demonstrates a swirling blood flow pattern with
color Doppler is most likely a _____.

15. An incomplete seal between the endograft and wall of the aorta may result in an _____. This may result in _____ or _____ of the aortic aneurysm.

16. Renal artery stenosis is most often a result of _____ and occurs at the _____ of the renal artery. Fibromuscular dysplasia causes renal artery stenosis less frequently, but these lesions are typically located in the _____ renal artery.

17. _____ _____ results from a lack of adequate blood supply to the intestinal tract causing postprandial pain, weight loss, and change in bowel habits.

18. Malignant invasion of the IVC most commonly occurs from _____ _____ _____. Respiratory changes are typically _____ or _____ below the level of obstruction.

19. _____ is a syndrome in which the IVC and/or one or more of the hepatic veins are occluded. In the primary form of the syndrome, the vessels are occluded by a congenital _____ _____, and in the secondary form they are occluded by _____ or _____.

20. While performing an examination of the liver, you have difficulty identifying the main portal vein; however, you do see multiple tortuous vessels in the region of the porta hepatis. This collateralization is called _____ _____ of the portal vein.

21. The normal portal vein measures less than _____ in diameter. In a patient with an acute portal vein thrombosis, the diameter of the portal vein may _____. With chronic thrombosis, the diameter may _____.

22. An increase in the portal venous pressure is called _____ _____. Common signs and symptoms include _____ and _____.

23. Portal hypertension can result in many sonographically visible changes including _____ varices, an enlarged _____ vein, and a patent _____ vein seen within the _____ _____ ligament.

24. Blood flow toward the liver is called _____, whereas blood flow away from the liver, as seen in some cases of portal hypertension, is called _____.

25. A TIPS, which stands for _____ _____ _____ _____, is used to decompress the portal vein pressure by connecting the _____ _____ with one of the _____ _____ bypassing flow through the liver.

Short Answer

1. While performing an abdominal sonogram to rule out renal artery stenosis, your patient asks you what the risk factors for atherosclerosis are and what are the signs and symptoms of atherosclerotic disease. How would you answer?

2. You are asked to perform a sonogram of the aorta to rule out an abdominal aortic aneurysm. What images would your protocol include and if an aneurysm was present, and what other vessels would you evaluate and why? What are some of the pitfalls to look out for when performing this examination?

3. What is the purpose of an aortic endograft? List the common complications of aortic endograft repair and describe the sonographic appearance of each complication.

4. Describe the two methods used to evaluate for renal artery stenosis sonographically. What measurements are taken for each method?

5. What are some of the common causes of portal hypertension in the United States? One of the common complications is the formation of collaterals. Where does this occur and why does it occur? What can be done to limit the symptoms of portal hypertension?

IMAGE EVALUATION/PATHOLOGY

Review the images and answer the following questions.

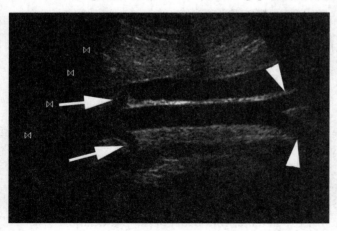

1. What vessels are the *arrows* pointing to? What vessels are the *arrowheads* pointing to? In what scanning plane would this image have to be acquired to view these vessels in this manner?

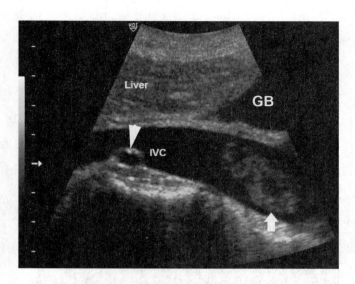

2. What is the *arrow* pointing to? What type of symptoms could this cause? What structure is the *arrowhead* pointing to?

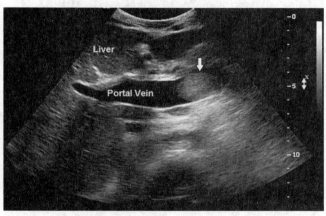

3. This image was obtained of the portal vein. What pathology is seen in this transverse sonogram of the portal vein? What is the normal measurement for the portal vein?

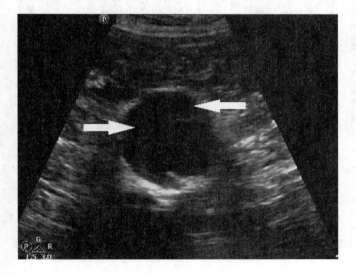

4. This image of the abdominal aorta was taken in the midline abdomen above the level of the umbilicus in an asymptomatic patient. What pathology is seen in this transvers sonogram? What are the *arrows* pointing to?

CASE STUDY

Review the images and answer the following questions.

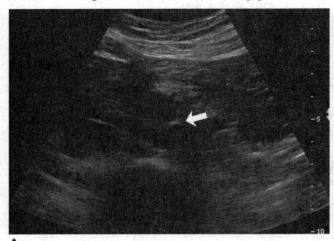

A

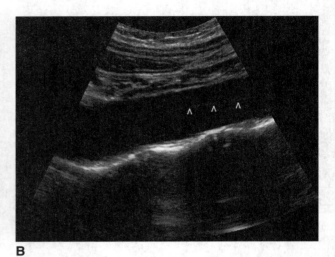

B

1. This patient was diagnosed with an aortic dissection. Review the following images of the aorta and right common iliac artery. What is the *arrow* pointing to on the transverse sonogram and the carets on the longitudinal sonogram? How would you confirm this diagnosis and ensure the findings were not artifacts?

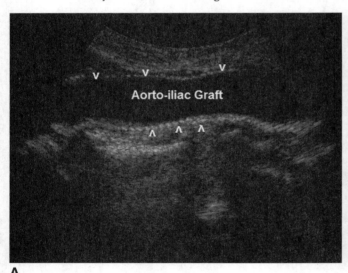

A

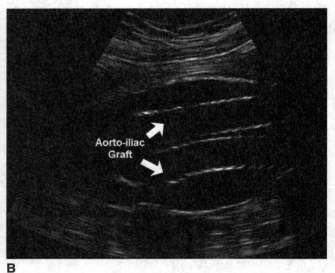

B

2. This patient presents for a sonography examination of the abdominal aorta. The patient was previously diagnosed with a large abdominal aortic aneurysm which was followed with an endovascular repair of the aneurysm (EVAR). What graft characteristics do the *carets* and *arrows* point identify within the lumen of the aorta? What is the normal measurement of the abdominal aorta?

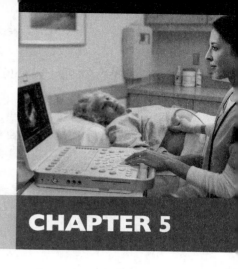

The Liver

CHAPTER 5

REVIEW OF GLOSSARY TERMS

Matching

Match the key terms with their definitions.

KEY TERMS

1. _____ AFP
2. _____ ALT
3. _____ AST
4. _____ contrast enhanced
5. _____ elastography
6. _____ falciform ligament
7. _____ Glisson capsule
8. _____ hepatofugal
9. _____ hepatomegaly
10. _____ hepatopetal
11. _____ jaundice
12. _____ ligamentum venosum
13. _____ ligamentum teres
14. _____ main lobar fissure
15. _____ porta hepatis
16. _____ Reidel lobe

DEFINITIONS

a. Remnant of ductus venosus seen as echogenic line separating caudate lobe from the left lobe
b. Fissure where the portal vein and hepatic artery enter the liver and the common hepatic duct exits
c. Tumor marker frequently elevated in cases of hepatocellular carcinoma and certain testicular cancers
d. Anatomic variant in which right lobe is enlarged and extends inferiorly
e. Technique uses ultrasound to assess stiffness of parenchyma
f. Blood flow toward the liver
g. Enlarged liver
h. Divides the right and left lobes of the liver; seen in sagittal plane as an echogenic line between the neck of the gallbladder and the main portal vein
i. Liver enzyme most specific to hepatocellular damage
j. Technique is useful in the evaluation of focal liver lesions
k. Yellowish pigmentation of the skin and whites of the eyes caused by increased levels of bilirubin in the blood
l. An enzyme found in all tissues but in largest amounts in the liver; increases with hepatocellular damage
m. Remnant of the left umbilical vein, seen in the transverse plane as a triangular echogenic foci dividing the medial and lateral segments of the left lobe of the liver
n. Fibroelastic connective tissue layer that surrounds the liver
o. Fold in the parietal peritoneum that extends from the umbilicus to the diaphragm and contains the ligamentum teres
p. Blood flow away from the liver

ANATOMY AND PHYSIOLOGY REVIEW

Image Labeling

Complete the labels in the images that follow.

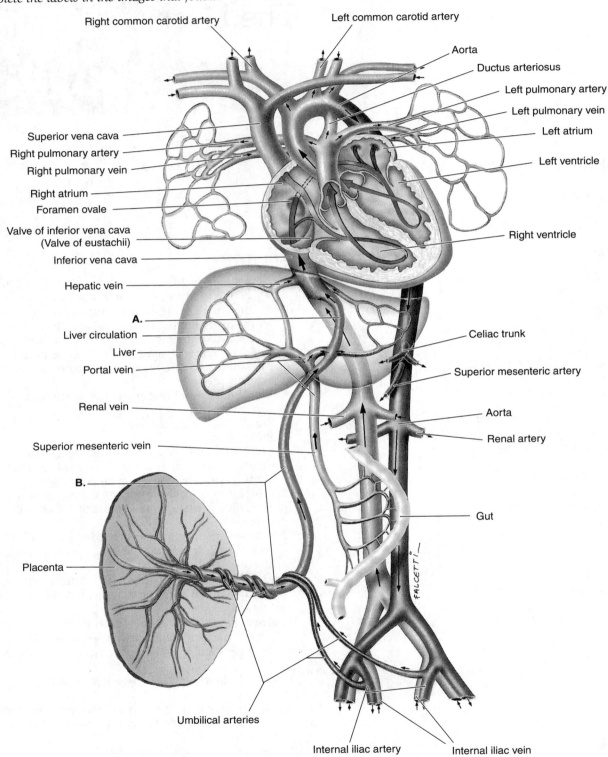

1. Fetal circulation

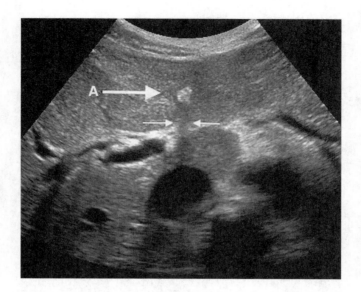

2. Liver anatomy

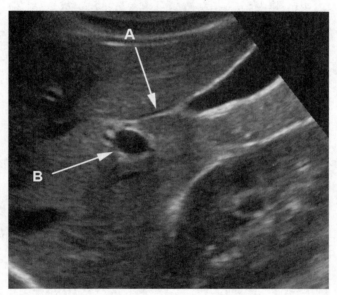

3. Liver anatomy

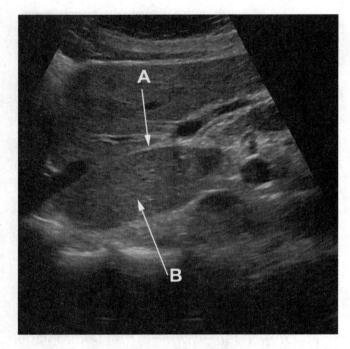

4. Liver anatomy

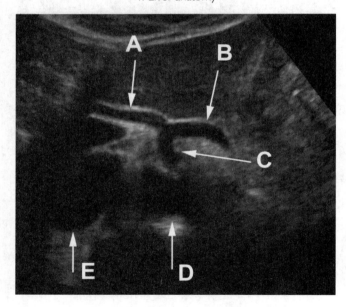

5. Vascular anatomy

CHAPTER REVIEW

Multiple Choice

Complete each question by circling the best answer.

1. **What is the normal liver length along the right surface?**
   a. 10 to 12 cm
   b. 11 to 14 cm
   c. 15 to 17 cm
   d. 19 to 22 cm

2. **What separates the left lobe from the caudate lobe?**
   a. ligamentum teres
   b. ligamentum venosum
   c. falciform ligament
   d. coronary ligament

3. Which of the following lies within the main lobar fissure?
   a. main portal vein
   b. right hepatic vein
   c. middle hepatic vein
   d. left hepatic vein

4. The anatomic quadrate lobe is what segmental division of the liver?
   a. lateral segment of the left lobe
   b. medial segment of the left lobe
   c. anterior segment of the right lobe
   d. posterior segment of the right lobe

5. If the sonographer is locating a mass within the right posterior segment of the liver, which vessel separates the right anterior liver segment from the right posterior liver segment?
   a. left hepatic vein
   b. middle hepatic vein
   c. right hepatic vein
   d. main portal vein

6. Which of the following statements differentiates between hepatic and portal veins?
   a. Hepatic veins have highly echogenic walls.
   b. Portal veins increase in caliber as they course away from the porta hepatis.
   c. Hepatic veins decrease in caliber as they course toward the diaphragm.
   d. Hepatic veins are intersegmental while portal veins are intrasegmental.

7. Which of the following are both interlobar and intersegmental?
   a. portal veins
   b. bile ducts
   c. hepatic veins
   d. hepatic arteries

8. Which of the following supplies oxygenated blood to the liver?
   a. portal vein
   b. hepatic artery
   c. hepatic veins
   d. hepatoduodenal artery

9. Which of the following is a liver function?
   a. concentration of bile
   b. secrete cholecystokinin
   c. production of clotting factors
   d. production of digestive enzymes amylase and lipase

10. What is the liver segment location for an echogenic mass consistent with a hemangioma if it is seen just anterior to the middle hepatic vein?
    a. posterior segment right lobe
    b. anterior segment right lobe
    c. medial segment left lobe
    d. lateral segment left lobe

11. Which of the following laboratory tests evaluates liver function?
    a. blood urea nitrogen
    b. mean corpuscular volume
    c. amylase
    d. alkaline phosphatase

12. What pathology should the sonographer look for specifically on an abdominal sonography examination on a patient with an indication of an elevated AFP?
    a. fatty infiltration
    b. polycystic liver disease
    c. hepatocellular carcinoma
    d. cavernous hemangioma

13. What is a typical characteristic of an intrahepatic mass?
    a. causes an anterior displacement of the right kidney
    b. displays internal displacement of the liver capsule
    c. causes an anterior shifting of the IVC
    d. displaces hepatic vessels

14. Which of the following is a diffuse liver disease?
    a. hepatoma
    b. hepatitis
    c. lipoma
    d. peliosis Hepatis

15. Which of the following statements regards fatty infiltration of the liver?
    a. Fatty infiltration is always diffuse.
    b. It is easier to visualize intrahepatic vessels.
    c. The right renal cortex appears hyperechoic compared to the liver parenchyma.
    d. Focal fatty infiltration may be mistaken for a liver mass.

16. A 65-year-old man presents with elevated liver function tests. The sonography examination reveals a shrunken, echogenic right lobe, a relatively enlarged caudate lobe, and the liver contour is irregular. What is the most likely diagnosis?
    a. acute hepatitis
    b. cirrhosis
    c. chronic hepatitis
    d. hepatocellular carcinoma

17. Which benign liver tumor commonly occurs in patients with glycogen storage disease?
    a. adenoma
    b. hepatoma
    c. hemangioma
    d. lipoma

18. If you are having trouble visualizing the posterior portion of the liver in a patient with fatty infiltration, which of the following may help?
    a. increasing the TGCs in the near field
    b. decreasing the overall gain
    c. decreasing the depth
    d. lowering the frequency

19. In focal fatty sparing, normal tissue appears more hypoechoic than the surrounding liver tissue and may be mistaken for a mass. What is the typical location for this to occur?
    a. dome of the liver
    b. posterior liver near the right kidney
    c. region of the porta hepatis near the gallbladder
    d. lateral segment of the left lobe

20. What does a person with cirrhosis have a higher incidence of developing?
    a. hepatoma
    b. cavernous hemangioma
    c. hepatic adenoma
    d. hepatic hemangiosarcoma

21. Which of the following may be seen in patients with late stage cirrhosis?
    a. attenuates less sound
    b. caudate lobe atrophy
    c. hepatofugal flow in the portal vein
    d. shrunken atrophic spleen

22. What is the most likely diagnosis when the sonographic appearance is a mother cyst containing multiple daughter cysts?
    a. hepatic abscess
    b. echinococcal cyst
    c. polycystic liver disease
    d. chronic hematoma

23. A 38-year-old woman presents postcholecystectomy with RUQ pain, fever, and an elevated white count. What is the most likely diagnosis if the sonography examination reveals an irregular, hypoechoic mass with posterior enhancement in the region of the porta hepatis?
    a. hematoma
    b. focal fatty sparing
    c. pyogenic abscess
    d. hepatocellular carcinoma

24. Patients with AIDS are at greater risk of acquiring which liver pathology?
    a. schistosomiasis
    b. cavernous hemangioma
    c. venous outflow obstruction
    d. fatty liver infiltration

25. What is the most likely diagnosis if a 30-year-old woman presents for an abdominal sonogram to rule out the presence of gallstones and the examination reveals a well-defined, 2 cm, solitary, echogenic mass in the posterior right lobe?
    a. hepatic metastases
    b. hepatocellular carcinoma
    c. cavernous hemangioma
    d. amebic abscess

26. What is the most likely diagnosis of a well-defined, highly echogenic liver mass in the right posterior segment with an artifact causing the portion of the diaphragm directly distal to the mass to appear discontinuous with the remainder of the diaphragm?
    a. hepatic adenoma
    b. hepatic lipoma
    c. cavernous hemangioma
    d. hepatoma

27. What is the most likely diagnosis for a 60-year-old man with a history of alcoholic cirrhosis, increasing abdominal girth, and jaundice with the sonography examination revealing ascites, multiple hyperechoic lesions seen throughout the liver, and a tumor within the portal vein?
    a. hepatic metastases
    b. hepatic adenomas
    c. hepatocellular carcinoma
    d. Karposi sarcoma

28. Which of the following would rule-out either a congenital or acquired hepatic cystic lesions?
    a. well defined with sharp posterior wall
    b. lateral wall refractive edge shadowing
    c. no internal echoes, anechoic
    d. distal acoustic shadowing

29. What is the most likely diagnosis on a patient with RUQ pain and a normal sonography examination except in the right liver lobe there is a single, well-circumscribed anechoic lesion with posterior enhancement?
    a. simple liver cyst
    b. polycystic liver disease
    c. hematoma
    d. cavernous hemangioma

30. What is a recanalized paraumbilical vein typically the result of?
    a. hepatitis
    b. portal hypertension
    c. liver metastases
    d. amebic abscess

31. Which of the following is a disadvantage of using contrast enhanced ultrasound?
    a. Ultrasound contrast is not nephrotoxic.
    b. Vascularity may be visible in septations or mural nodules.
    c. Two or three people are required to perform the study.
    d. Assist in liver mass biopsies of isoechoic lesions.

32. Which of the following is an advantage of using contrast enhanced ultrasound?
    a. It can be used on patients allergic to CT and MRI contrast agents.
    b. It requires an intravenous injection site.
    c. The continuous documentation requires large video clips.
    d. It requires an individual to inject while the sonographer scans.

33. What determines why contrast images are obtained at a lower acoustic pressure setting?
    a. lesion depth
    b. mechanical Index
    c. transient effects
    d. thermal Index

34. What is the main clinical indication for liver elastography?
    a. Measure nodular contour and irregularity.
    b. Evaluate morphologic changes.
    c. Determine extent of variability with interpretation.
    d. Staging the degree of fibrosis in cases of chronic liver disease.

Fill-in-the-Blank

1. The liver is surrounded by a fibrous capsule called _____ _____ and is located within the _____ cavity.

2. After birth, the ductus venosus closes to become the _____ _____ and the left umbilical vein becomes the _____ _____. Both are important as they can become recanalized with certain disease processes, most commonly _____ _____.

3. The anatomy of the liver can be classified by different methods. The anatomic division divides the liver into four lobes: the _____ lobe, _____ lobe, _____ lobe, and _____ lobe, based on _____ _____. The segmental division is based on the liver's _____.

4. The left intersegmental fissure divides the _____ lobe into _____ and _____ segments. The left _____ vein is a sonographic landmark of the left intersegmental fissure.

5. The _____ lobe may be enlarged in patients with a history of cirrhosis or Budd–Chiari syndrome. Enlargement of the caudate lobe may cause compression of the _____.

6. A 28-year-old woman presents for an abdominal sonogram and you notice that the right lobe appears enlarged and extends inferiorly toward the pelvis. The texture appears homogenous and is continuous with the remainder of the right lobe. The most likely diagnosis is a _____ _____.

7. The basic functional unit of the liver is the _____. These cells carry out most of the metabolic functions of the liver. The _____ cells, macrophages that are part of the reticuloendothelial system, help break down red blood cells.

8. An anatomical variation in which the liver and gallbladder are found on the left side of the abdomen and the spleen is found on the right side is called _____ _____.

9. The portal triad is made up of the _____ vein, _____ artery, and _____ _____.

10. A _____ array transducer is typically used to evaluate the liver but a _____ array transducer can be used to evaluate the anterior liver capsule for surface nodularity in suspected cases of cirrhosis.

11. Fatty infiltration is also called _____ and is commonly caused in the United States by _____ _____ and _____.

12. With fatty infiltration, the echogenicity of the liver is _____, while the acoustic penetration is _____.

13. Inflammation of the liver is called _____. In the acute form, the liver appears _____, causing the portal vessels to appear more _____.

14. The most common cause of cirrhosis in the United States is _____.

15. Patients with autosomal dominant polycystic kidney disease may also develop cysts in the _____, _____, and _____.

16. The majority of liver cysts are _____. Acquired cystic lesions of the liver may be the result of _____, _____, or _____ reactions.

17. The appearance of a liver hematoma will vary depending on the _____ of the bleed. Immediately following the injury, the hematoma will typically appear _____. Within a day, the hematoma may become _____; eventually clot forms and the hematoma becomes organized and complex. Chronic hematomas can become _____.

18. Hematomas are usually contained by the liver _____, although rupture can occur. A subcapsular hematoma will displace the liver _____ and have a _____ shape.

19. Echinococcal cysts are commonly referred to as _____ cysts. Rupture of an echinococcal cyst can result in _____ _____.

20. An amebic abscess is typically the result of parasites travelling to the liver from the _____ via the _____ _____.

21. Patients with HIV and AIDS are commonly infected by the organism _____ _____. When the liver is infected, sonographically the liver demonstrates a _____ _____ pattern.

22. The most common benign liver tumor is the _____.

23. Two benign liver lesions typically occur in women of childbearing age and have an association with oral contraceptive use. Those lesions are _____ _____ _____ and _____.

24. Hepatocellular carcinoma is also known as _____ and is the most common primary malignant liver tumor. In the United States, the most common predisposing factor is _____.

25. The liver function tests AST and ALT will be _____ with hepatocellular carcinoma and the tumor marker _____ is elevated in 70% of cases.

26. Hepatocellular carcinoma may invade the vasculature of the liver, including the _____ and _____ veins. Tumors may also cause biliary tract _____.

27. Liver _____ are much more common than primary liver tumors and can result from primary cancers of the _____, _____, _____, _____, _____, and _____.

28. Although liver metastases can have a wide range of sonographic appearances, metastases from colon cancer are typically _____, metastases from lung cancer typically have a _____ appearance, and lesions from lymphoma are typically _____.

29. Using the FDA approved ultrasound contrast, _____ _____ ultrasound can aid in the evaluation of liver lesions.

30. A sonogram obtained using elastogrpahy has areas of red in the ROI which is compatible with _____ _____.

Short Answer

1. Couinaud anatomy divides the liver into eight segments. How are these segments divided and what is the importance of this segmentation?

2. Imaging the entire liver sonographically sometimes requires creative techniques. Describe some of the techniques used to adequately image the liver.

3. In cases of cirrhosis, the caudate lobe is typically spared or enlarged. Why does this occur? In what other pathology is the caudate lobe enlarged?

4. The sonographer was asked to perform an abdominal sonogram to rule out cirrhosis in a patient with a history of alcohol abuse. What sonographic features will the sonographer look for to confirm the diagnosis?

5. The sonographer is evaluating a patient with a recent diagnosis of hepatocellular carcinoma. What are the clinical signs and symptoms of hepatocellular carcinoma? What might be seen sonographically?

IMAGE EVALUATION/PATHOLOGY

Review the images and answer the following questions.

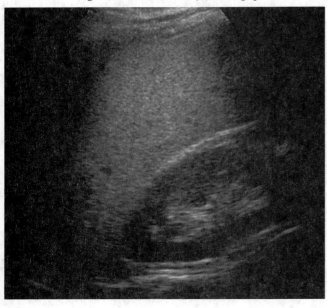

1. A 38-year-old man with a history of diabetes and obesity presents for an abdominal sonogram due to elevated LFTs. While performing the examination, the sonographer is having difficulty penetrating through the liver. Describe the liver seen in this image. What is the most likely diagnosis?

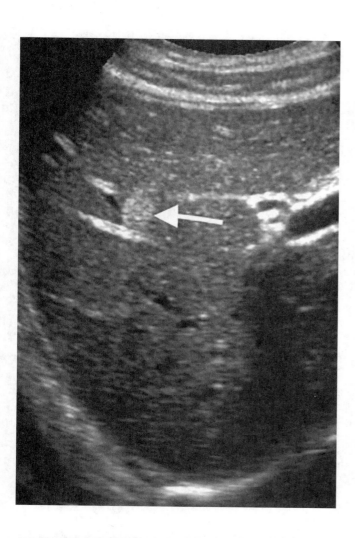

2. A 42-year-old woman presents for an abdominal sonogram with a history of gallbladder disease. While evaluating the right lobe of the liver, the sonographer located the finding seen in this image. Describe the appearance of the mass on the sonogram. What is the most likely diagnosis?

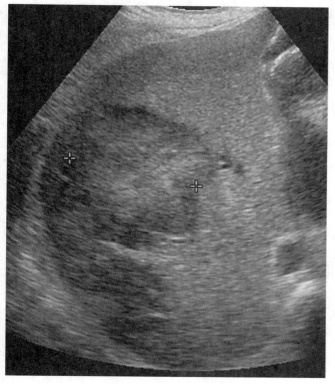

3. Provide a sonographic description of this mass. List three differential diagnoses for a mass with this appearance.

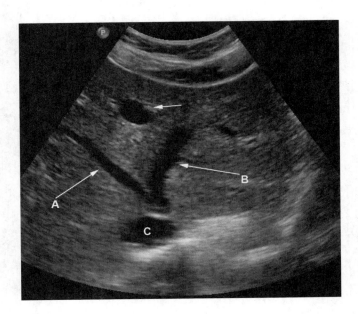

4. Identify the vessels labeled A, B, and C. In which liver segment is the simple cyst (*arrow*) located based on the vasculature?

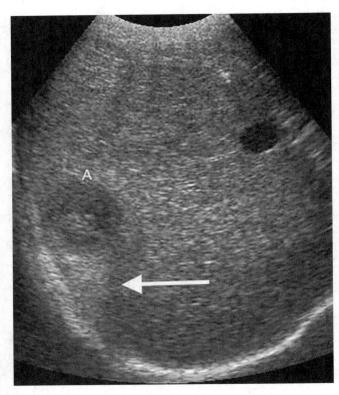

5. This sagittal scan represents a pyogenic liver abscess. What is seen in the abscess and what is the *arrow* pointing to? What type of clinical symptoms might this person be experiencing?

CASE STUDY

Review the images and answer the following questions.

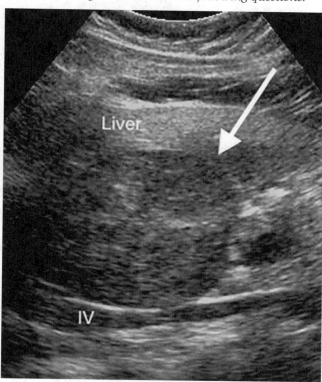

1. The 32-year-old female patient was referred to evaluate for gallstones. The laboratory tests were normal, a medical history is an 8-year history of oral contraceptive use, and recent intolerance for certain foods. Describe what is seen on the sonogram and give a possible diagnosis.

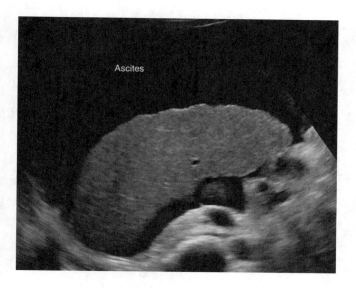

2. This is a transverse scan on a 57-year-old man with end-stage alcoholic liver disease. Describe what pathology is demonstrated on the sonogram?

The Gallbladder and Biliary System

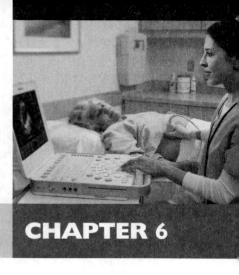

CHAPTER 6

REVIEW OF GLOSSARY TERMS

Matching

Match the key terms with their definitions.

KEY TERMS

1. _____ cholangitis

2. _____ cholecystectomy

3. _____ cholecystitis

4. _____ cholecystokinin

5. _____ choledocholithiasis

6. _____ common bile duct

7. _____ cystic duct

8. _____ cholelithiasis

9. _____ gallbladder

10. _____ pneumobilia

11. _____ sludge

12. _____ Phyrgian cap

13. _____ Murphy sign

14. _____ junctional fold

DEFINITION

a. Calculi located within the bile duct
b. Air within the bile ducts
c. Formation or presence of stones within the gallbladder
d. Hormone which stimulates gallbladder contraction
e. Fold within the neck or body of the gallbladder
f. Pain in the area of the gallbladder when pressure is applied by the ultrasound transducer
g. Inflammation of the bile ducts
h. Fold within the gallbladder fundus
i. Surgical removal of the gallbladder
j. Solid, semisolid, or thickened bile within the gallbladder or bile duct
k. Pear-shaped sac responsible for storing bile until it is released through the cystic duct
l. Duct which carries bile from the cystic and hepatic ducts to the duodenum
m. Acute or chronic inflammation of the gallbladder
n. Duct of the gallbladder which joins with the hepatic duct to form the common bile duct

ANATOMY AND PHYSIOLOGY REVIEW

Image Labeling

Complete the labels in the images that follow.

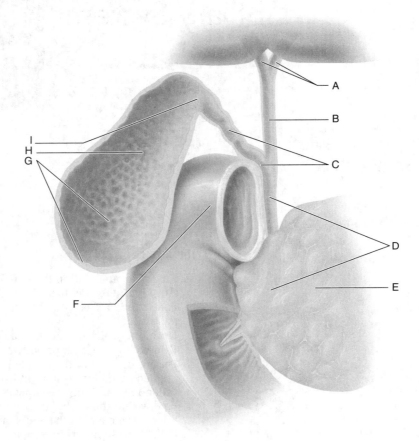

1. Biliary system

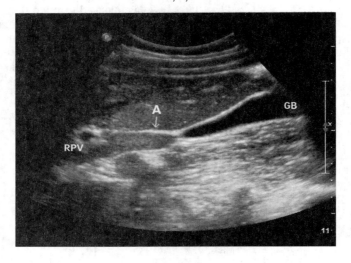

2. Anatomy

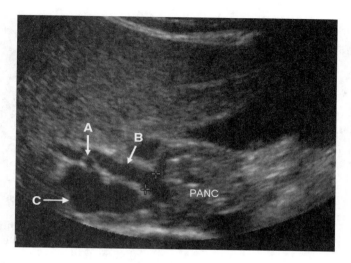

3. Porta hepatis

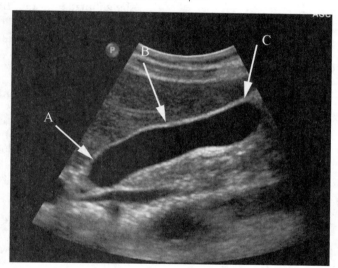

4. Gallbladder

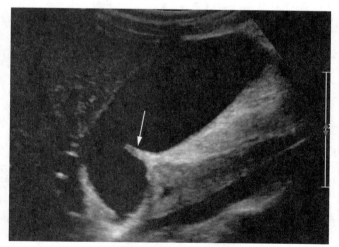

5. Anatomical variant

CHAPTER REVIEW

Multiple Choice

Complete each question by circling the best answer.

1. What is the upper limit of normal for the measurement of the gallbladder wall?
   a. 2 mm
   b. 3 mm
   c. 4 mm
   d. 5 mm

2. Which of the following is NOT included in the portal triad?
   a. hepatic vein
   b. hepatic artery
   c. portal vein
   d. bile duct

3. What is the normal measurement for an intrahepatic bile duct?
   a. less than 1 mm
   b. less than 2 mm
   c. less than 3 mm
   d. less than 4 mm

4. What is a fold or kinking of the gallbladder fundus onto the body commonly called?
   a. Hartman pouch
   b. valve of Heister
   c. Phrygian cap
   d. ampulla of Vater

5. Which of the following is the hormone that causes the gallbladder to contract and the sphincter of Oddi to relax, allowing bile to flow from the gallbladder to the small intestine?
   a. alkaline phosphatase
   b. bilirubin
   c. lactic dehydrogenase
   d. cholecystokinin

6. Which anatomical landmark can help locate a gallbladder that is difficult to visualize?
   a. main lobar fissure
   b. ligamentum venosum
   c. ligamentum teres
   d. coronary ligament

7. Which of the following is NOT a laboratory test that can be used to evaluate the biliary system?
   a. lipase
   b. alkaline phosphatase
   c. bilirubin
   d. lactic dehydrogenase

8. A 2-month-old infant presents with persistent jaundice and a palpable RUQ mass. The sonogram demonstrates a normal gallbladder and a cystic mass in the porta hepatis that appears to be separate from the gallbladder. The CBD appears to be entering the cystic mass. What is the most likely diagnosis?
   a. choledochal cyst
   b. interposition of the gallbladder
   c. biliary atresia
   d. multiseptate gallbladder

9. A 2-week-old infant presents with a sudden onset of jaundice. The sonogram demonstrates intrahepatic ductal dilatation but does not demonstrate a gallbladder or CHD. Which congenital biliary anomaly is the most likely cause?
   a. choledochal cyst
   b. interposition of the gallbladder
   c. biliary atresia
   d. mulitseptate gallbladder

10. Which of the following is NOT a symptom of gallbladder disease?
    a. nausea and vomiting
    b. epigastric or RUQ pain
    c. pain that radiates to the right shoulder
    d. hematuria

11. Which of the following statements regarding gallstones is FALSE?
    a. The prevalence of gallstones is higher in females than males.
    b. The majority of stones in the United States are made up of cholesterol.
    c. The majority of gallstones cause symptoms.
    d. Abnormal gallbladder emptying and altered absorption are precursors to stone formation.

12. Which of the following statements regarding gallbladder polyps is FALSE?
    a. Polyps will move to the dependent portion of the gallbladder with change in patient position.
    b. Polyps are attached to the gallbladder wall by a stalk.
    c. Polyps typically do not shadow.
    d. Polyps are typically adenomatous or made of cholesterol.

13. What is the most common malignancy to metastasize to the gallbladder?
    a. breast
    b. lung
    c. colon
    d. melanoma

14. A comet-tail reverberation artifact is seen originating from the anterior gallbladder wall. What gallbladder pathology is most likely causing this artifact?
    a. gallbladder carcinoma
    b. adenomyomatosis
    c. gallstone
    d. sludge

15. With a distal obstruction such as a mass in the head of the pancreas, which part of the biliary tree is the first to dilate?
    a. common bile duct
    b. common hepatic duct
    c. gallbladder
    d. intrahepatic duct

16. Which of the following will cause a thin-walled gallbladder?
    a. chronic cholecystitis
    b. acute cholecystitis

    c. a fatty meal
    d. hydrops

17. An abdominal sonogram demonstrates a large hypoechoic mass in the head of the pancreas. The gallbladder is enlarged with a thin wall. Murphy sign is negative. No gallstones are seen and the bile ducts are normal in caliber. What is the most likely diagnosis?
    a. cholelithiasis
    b. choledocholithiasis
    c. cholecystitis
    d. courvoisier gallbladder

18. A 76-year-old patient presents for an abdominal sonography examination with chronic abdominal pain. An irregular mass is seen projecting into the gallbladder lumen. Color Doppler detects flow within the mass. Gallstones are also seen. What is the most likely diagnosis?
    a. adenomyomatosis
    b. gallbladder carcinoma
    c. courvoisier gallbladder
    d. gallbladder sludge and stones

19. Which of the following does NOT increase a patient's risk of developing gallbladder malignancy?
    a. septate gallbladder
    b. chronic cholecystitis
    c. porcelain gallbladder
    d. cholelithiasis

20. Which of the following would cause intrahepatic dilation with a normal gallbladder and CBD?
    a. carcinoma in the pancreatic head
    b. gallstone in the gallbladder neck
    c. stone in the distal CBD
    d. Klatskin tumor

Fill-in-the-Blank

1. The normal distended gallbladder measures _____ cm in length and less than _____ cm in the AP and transverse dimensions.

2. Because the gallbladder lies within the _____ _____ _____ between the right and left hepatic lobes, this structure can be used as a landmark to locate a contracted gallbladder.

3. The gallbladder is divided into three sections: the _____, _____, and _____.

4. The right and left hepatic ducts join in the porta hepatis to form the _____ _____ _____, which is joined by the _____ _____ to form the common bile duct.

5. The purpose of the gallbladder is to _____ and _____ bile.

6. An infundibulum at the neck of the gallbladder where stones may collect is a variant called a _____ _____.

7. _____ bilirubin is typically elevated in cases of obstructive jaundice as can occur with choledocholithiasis; _____ bilirubin is typically elevated with liver disease and hemolytic anemia.

8. Low-level, nonshadowing echoes are seen layering along the dependent portion of the gallbladder. The echoes move along with a change in patient position. The most likely diagnosis is _____.

9. Care must be taken not to misdiagnose a polyp as a gallstone. Unlike gallstones, polyps should not produce an acoustic _____ and should not _____ when the patient changes position.

10. _____ are seen in up to 95% of cases of gallbladder carcinoma. Other risk factors include chronic _____ and _____ gallbladder, or calcification of the gallbladder wall.

11. _____ _____ may be used to look for internal vascularity in a suspected gallbladder mass and to distinguish sludge from a malignant mass.

12. The two most common hyperplastic cholecystoses are _____ and _____.

13. A gallbladder that is enlarged, thin-walled, and not tender that is caused by a mass in the pancreatic head obstructing the common bile duct is called _____ _____.

14. A _____ _____ is a distended gallbladder caused by an obstruction of the gallbladder neck or cystic duct.

15. Patients with biliary system obstruction typically present with symptoms of _____ _____, _____, _____, and elevated _____ or _____ _____.

16. Bile ducts should be measured from the _____ wall to the _____ wall, with a CBD measurement greater than _____ mm considered abnormal.

17. _____ _____ can help distinguish dilated ducts from hepatic vessels.

18. Stones within the bile ducts, called _____, are the most common pathology of the biliary tree.

19. Primary malignancy of the bile ducts is called _____.

20. The most common location for cholangiocarcinoma to occur is at the porta hepatis. This type of cholangiocarcinoma is called a _____ _____.

Short Answer

1. List two pitfalls that might cause a false-positive gallbladder examination and two pitfalls that could cause a false-negative gallbladder examination. Explain how each of your examples could cause an incorrect diagnosis.

2. Describe the protocol for a sonographic examination of the biliary tree. Include the patient preparation, patient positioning, and required images.

3. What techniques can the sonographer utilize to demonstrate acoustic shadowing with small gallstones?

4. Explain the difference between intrinsic and extrinsic gallbladder wall thickening and list three examples of each.

5. Describe the sonographic appearance, clinical symptoms, and cause of both Courvoisier gallbladder and gallbladder hydrops.

IMAGE EVALUATION/PATHOLOGY

Review the images and answer the following questions.

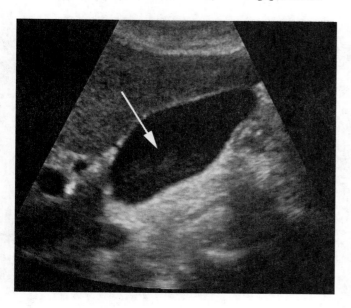

1. What pathology is the *arrow* pointing to in this image? What could you do to differentiate this pathology from a gallbladder mass?

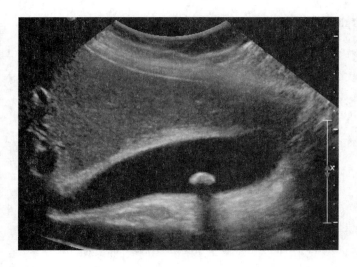

2. What pathology is demonstrated in this image? What criteria must be met for this pathology to be confirmed?

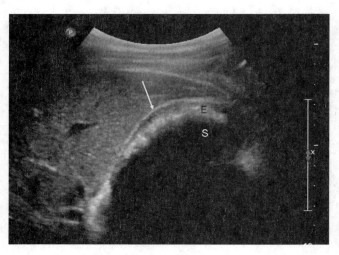

3. What pathology is seen in this image? Describe what you are seeing in this image.

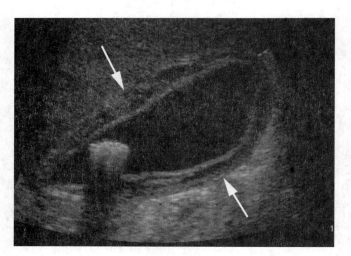

4. What are the *arrows* pointing to in this image? What is the normal measurement for this structure? What is the most likely diagnosis?

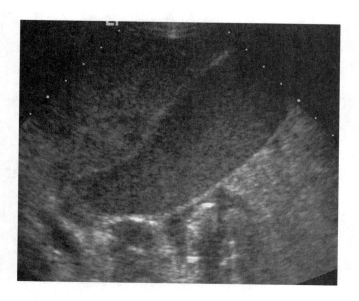

5. Describe the gallbladder seen in this image. What are some common causes of this pathology?

CASE STUDY

Review the images and answer the following questions.

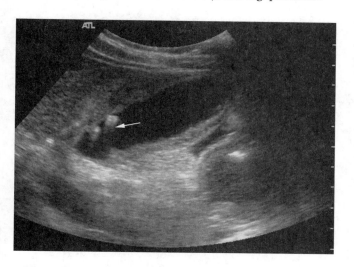

1. A 37-year-old woman presents for an abdominal sonography examination with a history of RUQ pain and intolerance to fatty foods. This sagittal image is taken of her gallbladder. What pathology do you see? What artifact is the *arrow* pointing to? How would you distinguish this pathology from gallstones?

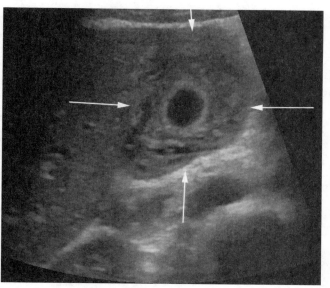

2. A 45-year-old man presents with a history of acute hepatitis, jaundice, and right upper quadrant pain. An examination of the upper abdomen is ordered to evaluate the liver and biliary system. This image was taken in the right upper quadrant. No gallstones were seen. What is the most likely diagnosis? What type of clinical symptoms does this pathology typically cause?

The Pancreas

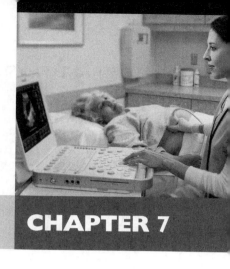

CHAPTER 7

REVIEW OF GLOSSARY TERMS

Matching

Match the terms with their definitions.

KEY TERMS

1. _____ acini cells

2. _____ alpha cells

3. _____ amylase

4. _____ beta cells

5. _____ delta cells

6. _____ endocrine

7. _____ exocrine

8. _____ glucagon

9. _____ insulin

10. _____ islets of Langerhans

11. _____ lipase

12. _____ pseudocyst

13. _____ phlegmon

14. _____ somatostatin

DEFINITION

a. Secreting into a duct
b. Performs endocrine function, secreting insulin
c. Fat-digesting enzyme
d. Performs exocrine function, secreting digestive enzymes
e. An abnormal cavity resembling a true cyst but not lined with epithelium
f. Performs endocrine function, secreting glucagon
g. Hormone secreted by delta cells, functions to regulate insulin and glucagon production
h. Enzyme that digests carbohydrates
i. Endocrine portion of the pancreas made up of alpha and beta cells that produce insulin and glucagon
j. Diffuse inflammatory reaction to infection spreading along fascial pathways, producing edema
k. Hormone secreted by the alpha cells, functions to increase activity of phosphorylase
l. Secreting into blood or tissue
m. Performs endocrine function, secreting somatostatin
n. Hormone secreted by beta cells, functions to increase uptake of glucose and amino acids

ANATOMY AND PHYSIOLOGY REVIEW

Image Labeling

Complete the labels in the images that follow.

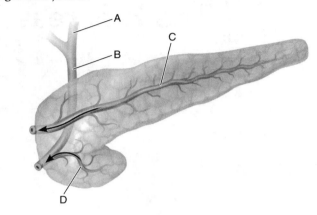

1. Pancreatic anatomy

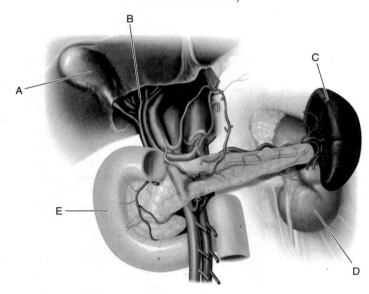

2. Surrounding anatomy

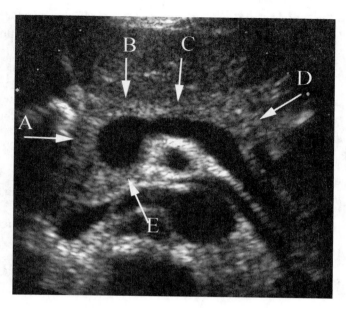

3. Pancreatic divisions

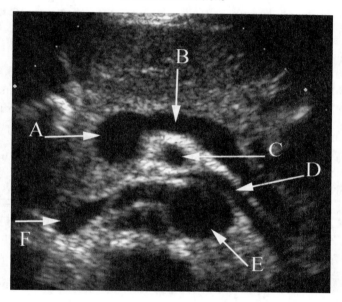

4. Vascular anatomy

CHAPTER REVIEW

Multiple Choice

Complete each question by circling the best answer.

1. Which of the following statements regarding the pancreas is FALSE?
   a. The pancreas is retroperitoneal.
   b. The pancreas is surrounded by a rigid capsule.
   c. The pancreas is made up of a head, neck, body, and tail.
   d. The pancreas is frequently obscured by bowel gas during sonographic examination.

2. Which portion of the pancreas is found anterior to the IVC and posterior to the superior mesenteric vein?
   a. uncinate process
   b. head
   c. neck
   d. body

3. Which portion of the pancreas lies just anterior to the portal confluence?
   a. uncinate process
   b. head
   c. neck
   d. body

4. Which of the following is a congenital anomaly of the pancreas in which the head of the pancreas surrounds the duodenum, frequently causing complete or partial duodenal stenosis or atresia?
   a. pancreatic divisum
   b. ectopic pancreas
   c. pancreatic pseudocyst
   d. annular pancreas

5. Which of the following produces insulin?
   a. alpha cells
   b. beta cells
   c. delta cells
   d. acini cells

6. Which laboratory values are used most often to diagnose pancreatic disease?
   a. BUN and creatinine
   b. WBC and RBC
   c. AST and ALT
   d. amylase and lipase

7. A normal main pancreatic duct located in the pancreatic head should not exceed what measurement?
   a. 1.5 mm
   b. 2.5 mm
   c. 3.5 mm
   d. 4.5 mm

8. In a transverse view of the pancreatic head, which vessel can be seen anterior to the CBD?
   a. gastroduodenal artery
   b. splenic vein
   c. hepatic artery
   d. superior mesenteric artery

9. Which of the following provides the best acoustic window to the pancreas?
   a. right lobe of the liver
   b. left lobe of the liver
   c. duodenum
   d. stomach

10. Which of the following techniques can aid in sonographic visualization of the pancreas?
    a. having the patient drink water to displace gas in the stomach
    b. imaging the pancreas at the start of the examination to reduce air in the stomach
    c. rotating the patient into the RLD position to visualize the tail of the pancreas
    d. all of the above may be used to image the pancreas

11. Which of the following statements regarding cystic fibrosis is FALSE?
    a. Cystic fibrosis can result in pancreatic insufficiency.
    b. Sonographically, the pancreas will appear hypoechoic and small.
    c. Liver and gallbladder disease are also common in children with cystic fibrosis.
    d. Children with cystic fibrosis may experience acute and chronic pancreatitis.

12. What are the two most common causes of acute pancreatitis?
    a. biliary tract disease and diabetes
    b. annular pancreas and cystic fibrosis
    c. alcohol abuse and diabetes
    d. biliary tract disease and alcohol abuse

13. In comparison to the normal pancreas, how does the pancreas in a patient with acute pancreatitis typically appear?
    a. smaller and more echogenic
    b. larger and more echogenic
    c. larger and more hypoechoic
    d. smaller and more hypoechoic

14. Where are pancreatic pseudocysts most often found?
    a. anterior to the pancreatic head
    b. posterior to the pancreatic body
    c. near the pancreatic tail
    d. lateral to the pancreatic head

15. Which of the following describes the sonographic appearance of chronic pancreatitis?
    a. a heterogeneously echogenic gland with calcifications seen throughout the parenchyma
    b. an enlarged hypoechoic gland with cystic formation
    c. a small hypoechoic gland with calcifications seen in the parenchyma
    d. chronic pancreatitis never affects the sonographic appearance of the pancreas

16. What is the most common malignant pancreatic tumor?
    a. cystadenocarcinoma
    b. adenocarcinoma
    c. squamous cell carcinoma
    d. insulinoma

17. Pancreatic adenocarcinomas typically occur in what portion of the pancreas?
    a. head
    b. neck
    c. body
    d. tail

18. What is the most common islet cell tumor?
    a. gastrinoma
    b. insulinoma
    c. glucogonoma
    d. cystadenoma

19. If a mass is detected in the pancreatic head what other organ should be evaluated?
    a. stomach
    b. duodenum
    c. gallbladder
    d. left kidney

20. What is the most common cystic lesion found within or near the pancreas?
    a. mucinous cystic adenoma
    b. microcystic adenoma
    c. polycystic disease of the pancreas
    d. pancreatic pseudocyst

Fill-in-the-Blank

1. The body of the pancreas lies anterior to the _____, _____ _____ artery, and _____ _____ vein.

2. The tail of the pancreas is bordered posteriorly by the _____ vein, anteriorly by the _____, and laterally by the left _____.

3. The main pancreatic duct is also called the _____ of _____. Enzymes secreted by the pancreas are transported through this duct, which joins with the distal _____ _____ _____ to empty into the _____.

4. The Islets of _____ are part of the _____ system, which releases hormones directly into the bloodstream.

5. Insulin is released by a _____ feedback mechanism, meaning that as blood glucose levels _____ above a certain level, insulin is secreted by the beta cells and as blood glucose levels _____, insulin secretion is decreased.

6. An imbalance between insulin secretion and the metabolic needs of the human body will result in _____.

7. The pancreas secretes enzymes which are essential to digestion and the absorption of vital nutrients. These enzymes include amylase, which breaks down _____; _____, which breaks down fats; and trypsinogen and chymotrypsinogen, which break down _____ into amino acids.

8. In children, the normal pancreas is more _____ than the adult pancreas because children tend to have less pancreatic fat than adults.

9. In most sonographic examinations the _____ and _____ of the pancreas can be adequately visualized; however, the pancreatic _____ is more difficult to visualize.

10. Water can be given to increase visualization of the pancreas during the sonographic examination. If water is given to the patient, the patient should be examined in the _____ position so that air in the stomach will rise above the fluid.

11. Clinically, a patient with acute pancreatitis will present with _____ pain, radiating to the _____. This pain is characteristically relieved when the patient _____.

12. In patients with acute pancreatitis, serum _____ increases quickly and returns to normal within 3 to 10 days after onset of symptoms, whereas serum _____ remains elevated longer.

13. In acute pancreatitis, the echotexture of the pancreas is _____ due to edema and the borders of the gland may appear _____. The _____ _____ may dilate due to obstruction.

14. Pancreatic _____, a common complication of acute pancreatitis, are encapsulated collections of the by products of the tissue destruction that occurs in severe disease.

15. _____ _____ is the result of repeated attacks of acute pancreatitis and leads to fibrosis, destruction, and atrophy of functioning pancreatic tissue.

16. Pancreatic cancer is the _____ leading cause of cancer-related deaths in the United States because early detection is _____.

17. Adenocarcinoma of the pancreas arises from the _____ tissues, whereas islet cell tumors are _____ in origin.

18. Islet cell tumors typically occur in the _____ or _____ of the pancreas and are often _____ in size.

19. _____ adenomas are benign cystic lesions that occur most frequently in the pancreatic head and contain multiple cysts of varying sizes, whereas _____ _____ adenomas are malignant lesions composed of larger cystic areas that are frequently found within the pancreatic tail.

20. _____ disease is an autosomal dominant disease that is characterized by multiple small cysts in the liver, kidneys, and, less commonly, the pancreas.

Short Answer

1. Describe the technique used to evaluate the pancreas sonographically. Include probe selection, probe placement, patient preparation, and tricks used to image a difficult-to-visualize pancreas.

2. Which portion of the pancreas is part of the endocrine system? What is the endocrine function of the pancreas? Which portion of the pancreas is part of the exocrine system? What is the exocrine function of the pancreas?

3. A 45-year-old patient presents with symptoms of acute pancreatitis. What laboratory values would help with this diagnosis and what changes would you expect in these values?

4. List four causes of acute pancreatitis. What complications can occur with acute pancreatitis?

5. A 60-year-old patient presents with a large hypoechoic mass in the head of the pancreas consistent with an adenocarcinoma. The gallbladder is noted to be extremely dilated. What is the mechanism for gallbladder dilation in this patient? What is this condition called?

IMAGE EVALUATION/PATHOLOGY

Review the images and answer the following questions.

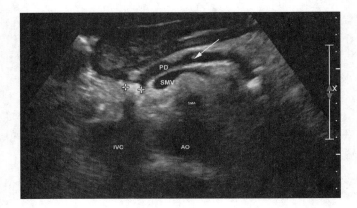

1. In this image, what are the calipers measuring? Where did this likely come from? The *arrow* is pointing to the main pancreatic duct. What is the normal measurement for this structure? Does this duct appear normal?

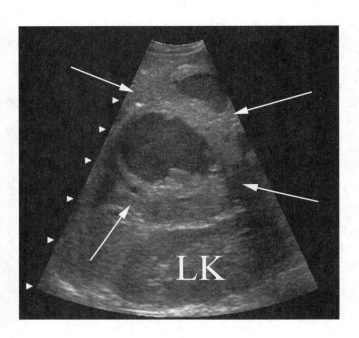

2. A 48-year-old patient with acute pancreatitis presents with worsening epigastric and left upper quadrant pain. The patient also has a fever and elevated amylase and lipase. This image is taken from the left upper quadrant. Describe what is seen in this image. What is the most likely diagnosis?

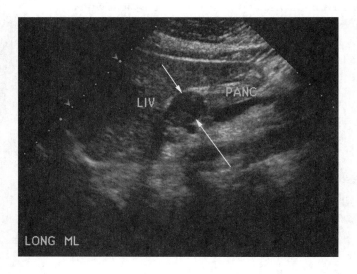

3. A 58-year-old patient presents with a history of indigestion and epigastric discomfort. This image was taken in the region of the pancreas. Describe the mass seen. Which solid pancreatic malignancy is more common in the pancreatic head?

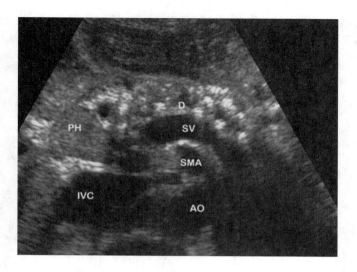

4. Describe the pancreas seen in this image. What is the most likely diagnosis? What are the most common causes of this pathology?

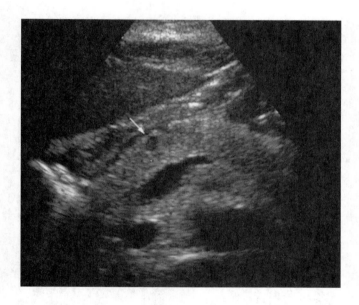

5. Describe the mass indicated by the *arrow*. Where in the pancreas is this mass located? What is the most likely diagnosis?

CASE STUDY

Review the images and answer the following questions.

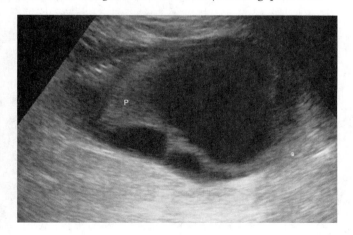

1. A 38-year-old patient with a history of chronic alcoholism presents with severe pancreatitis. This mass is seen in the left upper quadrant. Describe the mass. List some of the other possible complications from acute pancreatitis.

2. A 55-year-old patient presents with jaundice, weight loss, and difficulty eating. These sonographic images are taken of the pancreas. In the first image, what structures are indicated by the *arrows* A, B, and C? The next two images are sagittal images of the pancreatic head. Describe what is seen. What is the most likely diagnosis? What other structures will you evaluate for pathology based on these findings?

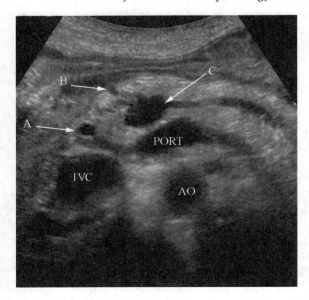

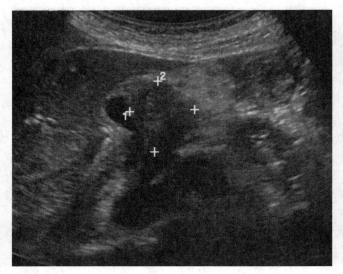

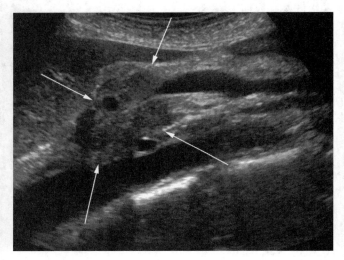

The Spleen

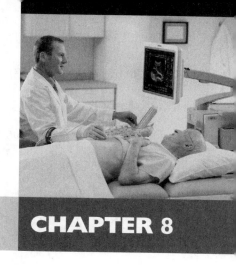

REVIEW OF GLOSSARY TERMS

Matching

Match the key terms with their definitions.

KEY TERMS

1. _____ erythrocyte

2. _____ erythropoiesis

3. _____ hematocrit

4. _____ infarct

5. _____ leukocyte

6. _____ leukocytosis

7. _____ leukopenia

8. _____ phagocytosis

9. _____ splenomegaly

DEFINITION

a. Tissue death caused by an interruption of the blood supply

b. Decreased white blood cell count, possibly the result of viral infection or leukemia

c. Red blood cell; contains hemoglobin

d. White blood cell; protects and fights against infection in the body

e. Elevated white blood cell count, usually due to infection

f. Process used by the red pulp to destroy old red blood cells

g. Enlarged spleen

h. Laboratory value of the percentage of blood volume made up of red blood cells

i. Process of red blood cell production

ANATOMY AND PHYSIOLOGY REVIEW

Image Labeling

Complete the labels in the images that follow.

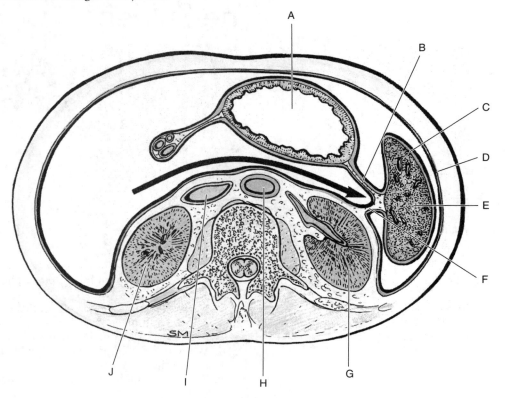

1. Relational anatomy

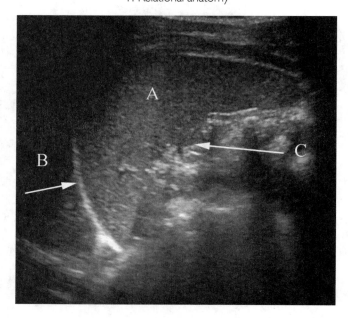

2. Splenic anatomy

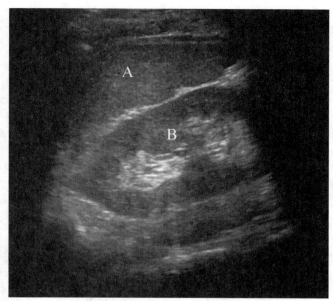

3. Anatomy of the left upper quadrant

CHAPTER REVIEW

Multiple Choice

Complete each question by circling the best answer.

1. Which of the following statements regarding the anatomy of the spleen is FALSE?
   a. The spleen is surrounded by a fibrous capsule.
   b. The spleen is a retroperitoneal organ.
   c. The spleen is located in the left hypochondrium.
   d. The spleen lies posterior to the stomach.

2. Which of the following ligaments does NOT help stabilize the spleen?
   a. falciform ligament
   b. lienorenal ligament
   c. gastrosplenic ligament
   d. phrenicocolic ligament

3. The spleen is considered enlarged when its length is greater than what measurement?
   a. 9 cm
   b. 11 cm
   c. 13 cm
   d. 15 cm

4. The splenic artery branches off which artery to supply blood to the spleen?
   a. aorta
   b. superior mesenteric
   c. pancreatic
   d. celiac axis

5. While scanning the spleen, you notice a small round mass that appears to be separate from the spleen in the region of the splenic hilum. The echotexture of the mass is similar to that of the spleen. What is the most likely diagnosis?
   a. splenic metastases
   b. accessory spleen
   c. splenic hemangioma
   d. ruptured spleen

6. While performing an abdominal sonography, you are having difficulty locating the spleen in its normal location in the left upper quadrant. As you scan the entire left side, you locate what appears to be the spleen in the left lower quadrant. What is the most likely explanation for this finding?
   a. asplenia
   b. accessory spleen
   c. situs inversus
   d. wandering spleen

7. A wandering spleen is at an increased risk of acquiring which of the following conditions?
   a. splenic rupture
   b. torsion and infarction
   c. splenomegaly
   d. leukemia and lymphoma

8. Which of the following statements regarding the function of the red pulp is FALSE?
   a. The red pulp is responsible for erythropoiesis throughout our lives.
   b. In cases of severe hemorrhage, the red pulp may release its reservoir into the bloodstream.
   c. Red pulp is responsible for the removal of worn-out red blood cells.
   d. The red pulp removes defective cells such as sickle and thalassemic cells from circulation.

9. Leukocytosis is the typical response to which of the following conditions?
   a. lupus erythematosus
   b. chemotherapy
   c. bacterial infection
   d. hemorrhage

10. What is leukopenia?
    a. a normal finding
    b. the result of severe inflammation
    c. frequently a side effect of chemotherapy
    d. an increase in the number of white blood cells in circulation

11. What is the normal echogenicity of the spleen?
    a. heterogeneous
    b. isoechoic to the liver
    c. hyperechoic to the liver
    d. hypoechoic to the liver

12. What is the most common sonographically visualized abnormality of the spleen?
    a. splenic rupture
    b. splenic abscess
    c. splenomegaly
    d. lymphoma

13. What is the most common cause of splenomegaly?
    a. mononucleosis
    b. lymphoma
    c. sickle cell anemia
    d. portal hypertension

14. While scanning the spleen, you notice multiple enlarged tortuous vessels in the splenic hilum. Color Doppler confirms that they are vascular in nature. Dilated vessels are also noted within the splenic parenchyma. What is the most likely cause of these findings?
    a. portal hypertension with collateral varices
    b. lymphoma with metastases
    c. splenic rupture with bleeding outside the capsule
    d. accessory spleen near the splenic hilum

15. Sonographically what is the splenic echogenicity when splenomegaly occurs?
    a. Does not change.
    b. Always becomes more hypoechoic.
    c. Always becomes more hyperechoic.
    d. Could be hyperechoic or hypoechoic but does not correlate with the cause of the enlargement.

16. Which of the following is NOT included as a focal lesion of the spleen?
    a. cysts
    b. infarcts
    c. splenomegaly
    d. granulomas

17. A patient with sickle cell disease presents for an abdominal sonogram complaining of recent left upper quadrant pain. A hypoechoic wedge shaped lesion is seen in the spleen. What is this typical of?
    a. lymphoma
    b. splenic rupture
    c. splenomegaly
    d. splenic infarct

18. A 10-year-old patient presents for an abdominal sonogram following blunt abdominal trauma that occurred during a bicycle accident. Which of the following would be an unusual finding in this patient?
    a. subcapsular hematoma
    b. free fluid in the peritoneum
    c. hematoma within the splenic parenchyma
    d. varices in the splenic hilum

19. Splenic calcifications usually result from which disease?
    a. splenomegaly
    b. lymphocytic
    c. angiosarcomas
    d. granulomatous

20. Which of the following may cause a small, shrunken spleen?
    a. mononucleosis
    b. acquired immunodeficiency syndrome
    c. sickle cell anemia
    d. portal hypertension

Fill-in-the-Blank

1. The spleen is located in the _____ cavity and is covered by peritoneum except at the splenic _____.

2. The spleen is located posterior to the _____, lateral to the _____ _____, _____ _____ _____, and _____ tail, and anterior to the _____.

3. Three ligaments help hold the spleen in its position in the left upper quadrant. The _____ ligament attaches the spleen to the left kidney. The _____ ligament attaches the spleen to the stomach and the _____ ligament, although not directly attached to the spleen, helps support its inferior end.

4. The average spleen measures _____ cm in length, _____ cm in width, and _____ cm in thickness.

5. A fibrous capsule surrounds the spleen and _____ project from the capsule into the organ, dividing the spleen into several compartments.

6. The spleen is made up of _____ and _____ pulp. The _____ pulp is composed of lymphatic tissue and the _____ pulp is composed of venous sinuses capable of storing more than 300 mL of blood.

7. The splenic vein joins with the _____ _____ _____ and can be seen posterior to the tail and body of the pancreas. Posterior to the _____ of the pancreas, the splenic vein joins with the _____ _____ _____ to form the main portal vein.

8. _____ is a very rare condition that leads to a congenital absence of the spleen.

9. Following a splenectomy, an _____ _____ may enlarge and assume the functions of the removed spleen.

10. The red pulp is responsible for _____ the peripheral blood. These functions include removal of _____ or _____ blood cells and the storage of _____.

11. The removal of defective and worn-out red blood cells occurs in the cords of _____.

12. The white pulp is part of the _____ system as it is a source of lymphocytes, macrophages, and antibodies. In addition, the white pulp can _____ bacteria that have bypassed the lymph nodes.

13. When imaging the spleen in the sagittal plane, views should always include the left _____ to evaluate for ascites or pleural fluid and the interface with the _____ _____.

14. The most common varice to occur in cases of portal hypertension is the _____ collateral, which diverts blood from the splenic vein to the _____ _____ vein and finally into the _____.

15. The most common malignant disease that affects the spleen is _____. Sonographically, _____ may be present if the spleen is diffusely infiltrated.

16. Acquired splenic cysts are _____, _____, or _____ in origin.

17. Patients who are _____ are more susceptible to fungal and bacterial abscesses of the spleen.

18. Patients with splenic infarcts are at risk for splenic _____. Signs to watch out for include increasing _____ hemorrhage, free _____ blood, and expanding _____ area within the infarct.

19. In patients with both Hodgkin disease and non-Hodgkin lymphoma, the spleen may contain focal _____ or _____ masses, may exhibit diffuse _____, or may appear sonographically _____.

20. The most common benign vascular lesion of the spleen is the _____.

Short Answer

1. The red pulp and white pulp that make up the spleen each have different functions. Describe the function of each and how they can be affected by pathological processes.

2. You are asked to perform an abdominal sonogram to rule out splenomegaly. What are the most common causes of splenomegaly and how does the anatomy of the spleen allow for such an increase in size?

3. Your patient presents with a history of bacterial endocarditis now complaining of left upper quadrant pain, fever, and leukocytosis. Splenic abscess is suspected. Describe the sonographic appearance of splenic abscess. What characteristics can help confirm the diagnosis?

4. The spleen is the most frequently damaged organ in blunt abdominal trauma. Why is the spleen so commonly injured? Describe the appearance of spleen in a trauma situation.

5. The spleen is commonly affected in patients with sickle cell anemia. Describe the variation in sonographic appearance that can occur with this disease.

IMAGE EVALUATION/PATHOLOGY

Review the images and answer the following questions.

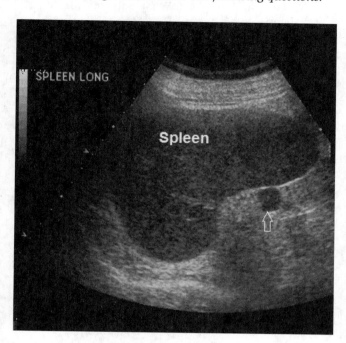

1. What structure is the arrow pointing to in this image? What is the significance of this structure?

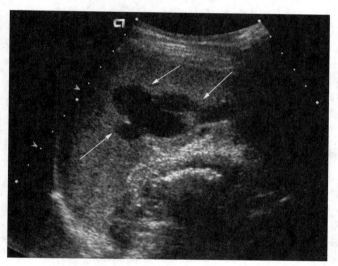

2. A 10-year-old girl presents for a sonogram of the spleen following a bicycle accident. Describe what is seen in this sagittal image of the spleen. What is the most likely diagnosis? What other areas in the abdomen will you evaluate based on these findings? Which lab value may be associated with this finding?

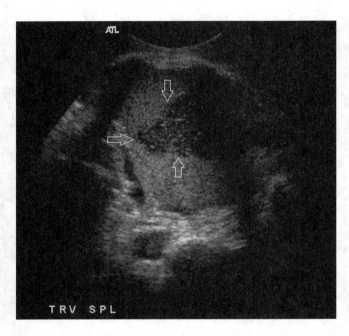

3. A 12-year-old patient with a history of sickle cell disease presents in a sickle cell crisis with severe left upper quadrant pain. Describe what is seen in this image of the spleen. What is the most likely diagnosis?

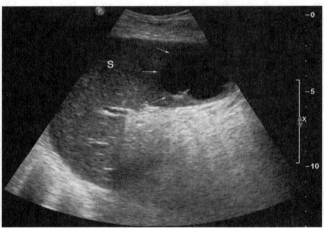

4. Describe what is seen in this image of the spleen. List three of the most common causes of this splenic pathology.

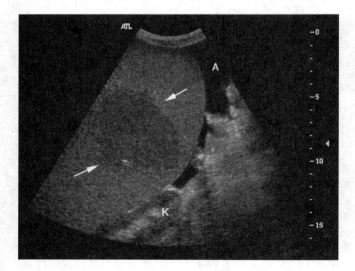

5. A 54-year-old patient presents with a history of lymphoma. Describe what is seen in this image of the spleen. What is the typical appearance of the spleen in a patient with lymphoma?

CASE STUDY

Review the images and answer the following questions.

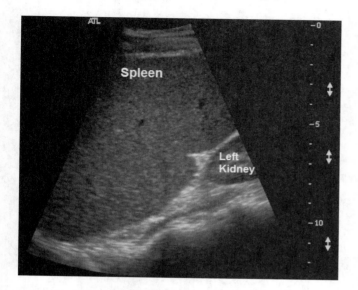

1. A 47-year-old man presents for an abdominal sonogram with a history of chronic alcohol abuse and cirrhosis. What pathology is seen in this image of the spleen? What is the normal measurement of the spleen? Why does the spleen enlarge in cases of liver cirrhosis? You are asked to evaluate the splenic hilum with color Doppler. What are you looking for?

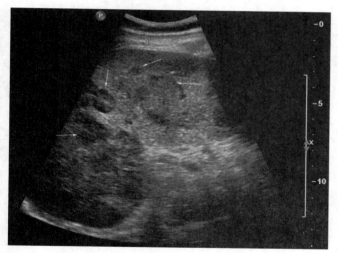

2. A 56-year-old woman presents with a history of pancreatic cancer. Describe what is seen in this image of the spleen. What is the most likely diagnosis? What other pathology may cause multiple target or hypoechoic lesions in the spleen?

The Gastrointestinal Tract

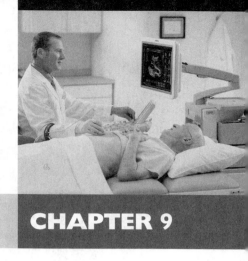

REVIEW OF GLOSSARY TERMS

Matching

Match the key terms with their definitions.

KEY TERMS

1. _____ appendicolith

2. _____ dysphagia

3. _____ ileus

4. _____ peristalsis

5. _____ ulcer

6. _____ volvulus

DEFINITION

a. Failure of the intestine to propel its contents due to diminished motility

b. Abnormal twisting of the intestines that can lead to obstruction, gangrene, perforation, and peritonitis

c. Difficulty swallowing

d. Fecalith or calcification found in the appendiceal lumen

e. An erosion in the mucosal layer of the wall of the GI tract

f. Rhythmic dilatation and contraction that propels the contents of the GI tract

ANATOMY AND PHYSIOLOGY REVIEW

Image Labeling

Complete the labels in the images that follow.

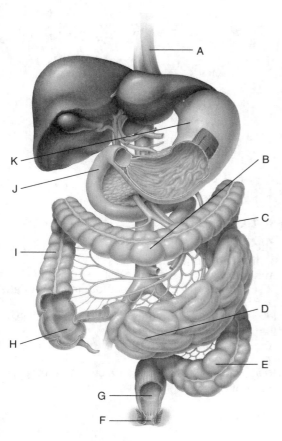

1. Gastrointestinal tract

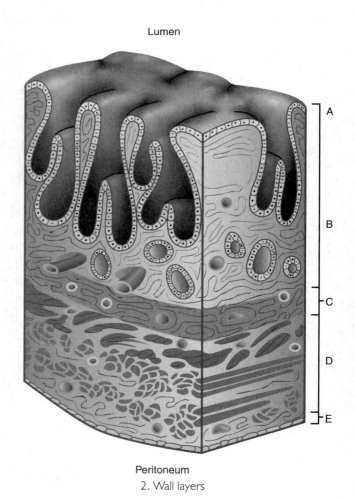

Lumen

Peritoneum

2. Wall layers

CHAPTER REVIEW

Multiple Choice

Complete each question by circling the best answer.

1. Which of the following is NOT a layer of the bowel wall?
   a. lamina propria
   b. intima media
   c. muscularis mucosa
   d. serosa

2. What is the innermost layer of the bowel wall?
   a. epithelium
   b. serosa
   c. intima
   d. muscularis

3. What is the most common esophageal cancer most commonly located in the upper and mid-esophagus.
   a. squamous cell
   b. lymphoma
   c. adenocarcinoma
   d. leiomyosarcoma

4. Which of the following describes the location of the esophagogastric junction?
   a. posterior to the left lobe and to the right of the abdominal aorta
   b. posterior to the left lobe and posterior to the abdominal aorta
   c. posterior to the left lobe and anterior to the aorta
   d. the esophagogastric junction can never be visualized sonographically

5. Where are the layers of the GI tract wall thickest?
   a. esophagus
   b. stomach
   c. small intestine
   d. large intestine

6. What should the bowel wall measure when the stomach is not distended?
   a. 1 to 4 mm
   b. 2 to 4 mm
   c. 4 to 6 mm
   d. 3 to 8 mm

7. Where does inflammation start in Crohn disease?
   a. Muscularis mucosa
   b. Muscularis propria
   c. Serosa
   d. Submucosa

8. Your patient has been referred for an abdominal sonography examination with a history of abdominal pain and Crohn disease. Which of the following does Crohn disease primarily affect?
   a. ileum
   b. duodenum
   c. stomach
   d. cecum

9. Which of the following statements regarding the jejunum and ileum is FALSE?
   a. The jejunum and ileum lie to the right and left of the abdomen, respectively.
   b. The valvulae conniventes of the mucosa can usually be seen if fluid is present within the loops.
   c. The diameter of the jejunum and ileum should measure less than 3 cm.
   d. Peristalsis should be visualized in the normal small bowel.

10. Which of the following CANNOT cause an ileus?
    a. surgery
    b. spinal fracture
    c. intussusception
    d. acute pancreatitis

11. A 2-year-old patient presents with abdominal pain and a palpable abdominal mass. Sonographically, an echogenic mass is seen in the midline and in the transverse plane it appears to demonstrate multiple concentric rings. What is the most likely diagnosis?
    a. duodenal ulcer
    b. pyloric stenosis
    c. crohn disease
    d. intussusception

12. What is the most common benign tumor of the small bowel?
    a. adenoma
    b. lipoma
    c. leiomyoma
    d. lymphoma

13. When performing a sonography examination, what structure will help locate the appendix?
    a. cecum
    b. duodenum
    c. jejunum
    d. urinary bladder

14. What term describes to a positive sign to rebound tenderness and pain located over the area of the appendix?
    a. Murphy sign
    b. McBurney sign
    c. McDowell sign
    d. McGinnty sign

15. Which of the following statements regarding appendicitis is FALSE?
    a. A calcified appendicolith can help identify an inflamed appendix.
    b. An inflamed appendix will demonstrate hyperemic flow with color or power Doppler.
    c. A noncompressible appendix greater than 6 mm is considered abnormal.
    d. Sonography cannot visualize a normal appendix.

16. A 20-year-old patient presents with right lower quadrant pain. The sonogram demonstrates an 8-mm noncompressible target shaped lesion at the area of maximum tenderness. A calcification is seen within the lesion. What is the most likely diagnosis?
    a. Crohn disease
    b. appendicitis with appendicolith
    c. intussusception with bowel tumor
    d. ileus with bowel distention

17. Where do the majority of colon cancers occur?
    a. sigmoid colon
    b. ascending colon
    c. cecum
    d. rectum and rectosigmoid colon

18. Your patient complains of abdominal pain; while scanning over the area of tenderness, you locate a loop of bowel with visible haustra. This is characteristic of which part of the GI tract?
    a. stomach
    b. small intestine
    c. large intestine
    d. all parts of the GI tract display this characteristic feature

19. Which part of the GI tract can be seen curving around the pancreatic head?
    a. stomach
    b. duodenum
    c. jejunum
    d. ileum

20. A patient presents with abdominal pain and your evaluation reveals multiple dilated fluid-filled small-bowel loops with markedly increased peristalsis. What is the most likely diagnosis?
    a. intussusception
    b. Crohn disease
    c. bowel obstruction
    d. diverticulitis

Fill-in-the-Blank

1. Sonography is not often the examination of choice for evaluating the GI tract due to the difficulty caused by the presence of _____ in the GI tract.

2. Both _____ and _____ approaches may be used to evaluate the GI tract sonographically.

3. Sonographically, the bowel wall is described as _____ layers. The layers are the innermost echogenic layer representing the _____ interface. Next is a hypoechoic layer made up of the _____, _____ _____, and _____ _____. Next is the echogenic _____, followed by the hypoechoic _____ _____, and finally the echogenic _____.

4. Squamous cell carcinoma can present with the clinical symptom of _____, or difficulty swallowing.

5. The fundus of the stomach lies _____ to the spleen and _____ to the left kidney. The body and antrum lie anterior to the _____.

6. Chronic gastritis may present with generalized thickening of the hypoechoic _____ layer of the stomach wall.

7. Gastric peptic ulcers are much less common than _____ ulcers in the United States, typically appearing along the antral portion of the _____ _____.

8. The folds that can sometimes be seen projecting into the fluid-filled lumen of the small bowel are called
   _____ _____.

9. Sonographically, the small bowel is typically more distended with an _____ than with an ileus.

10. With ileus, the small bowel is distended with _____ or _____, and peristalsis can be normal
    to _____ _____.

11. A volvulus will appear as a dilated, _____-shaped loop containing only _____ and no air.

12. Intussusception is more common in _____ than in _____ When it does occur in adults, it is
    almost always secondary to a bowel _____.

13. Crohn disease is a common cause of bowel wall inflammation and presents sonographically as _____
    of the bowel wall and surrounding _____. The typical sonographic appearance is a _____
    _____ lesion.

14. The normal appendix extends from the _____ and should measure no more than _____ mm
    in diameter with a wall thickness of _____ mm or less.

15. The appendix is located under _____ point, which is located by drawing an imaginary line from the
    right anterosuperior _____ _____ to the umbilicus. The appendix is usually found at the
    midpoint of this line.

16. When evaluating the appendix, the sonographer should use the _____ _____ technique to
    displace gas- or fluid-filled bowel loops and locate the area of maximum tenderness.

17. Complications of appendicitis include _____ formation, _____, or _____.

18. Lymphadenopathy in the right lower quadrant surrounding the cecum is termed _____
    _____. Lymph nodes greater than _____ mm are considered abnormal.

19. The colon lies along the _____ of the abdomen, is larger in diameter than the small bowel, and contains
    characteristic _____ folds. When the colon is not distended, the wall should measure _____
    mm thick.

20. Ulcerative colitis is an inflammatory disease that affects the _____ and _____ layers of the
    colon. Inflammation starts in the _____ and may extend throughout the colon.

Short Answer

1. Although the majority of evaluations of the GI tract are performed transabdominally, endoluminal examinations
   can provide useful information. What structures can be evaluated with an endoluminal examination, and how does
   it compare to a transabdominal examination?

2. What techniques may be used to evaluate the stomach and duodenum sonographically?

3. You are asked to perform an abdominal sonogram to rule out appendicitis in a 10-year-old patient. Describe the technique used to locate and evaluate the appendix for appendicitis.

IMAGE EVALUATION/PATHOLOGY

Review the images and answer the following questions.

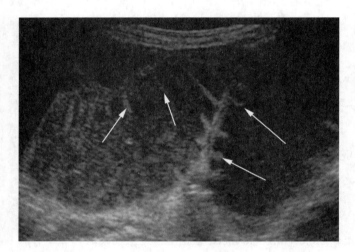

1. A 45-year-old patient presents with acute pancreatitis, abdominal pain, and distention. Peristalsis is noted within the bowel and is mildly increased. Describe the image shown. What is a possible diagnosis? What normal structures are the *arrows* pointing to?

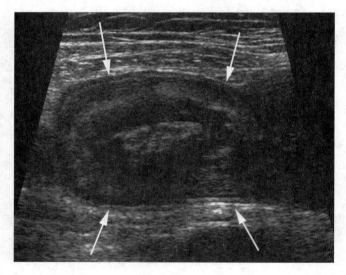

2. A 59-year-old patient presents for an abdominal sonogram with severe epigastric pain. The patient is able to demonstrate an area that is the most painful. This image is taken at that area. Multiple concentric rings are demonstrated within the visualized bowel. This is diagnostic of what bowel pathology? In adults, what is the most common cause of this pathology?

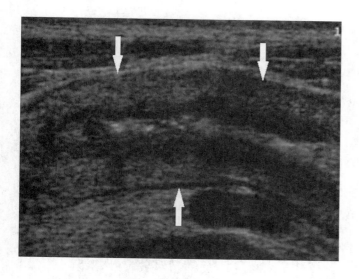

3. A 24-year-old patient presents with a history of Crohn disease. Describe the bowel seen in this image. Which part of the bowel is most commonly affected by Crohn disease?

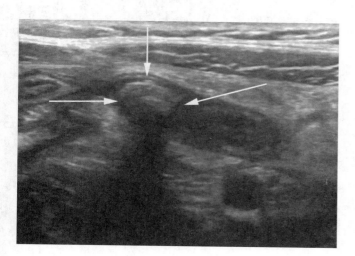

4. A 14-year-old patient presents with severe RLQ pain, nausea and vomiting, and leukocytosis. Your examination of the RLQ reveals this image. What are the *arrows* pointing to? What is the normal measurement for the wall of the appendix? What is the normal diameter of the appendix?

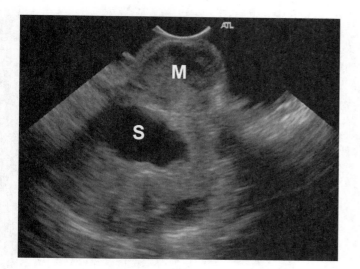

5. Describe what is seen in this image of the stomach. In what layer of the stomach wall do gastric carcinomas typically occur?

CASE STUDY

Review the images and answer the following questions.

1. A 6-year-old patient presents with RLQ pain and fever. These images are taken in the RLQ. Describe what is seen. What is the diagnosis? What complications may occur with this pathology?

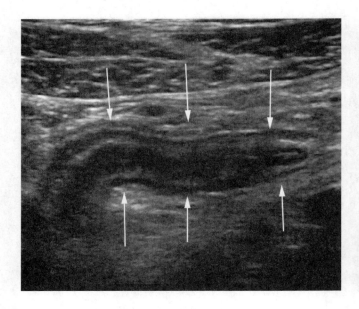
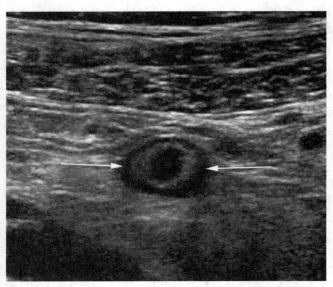

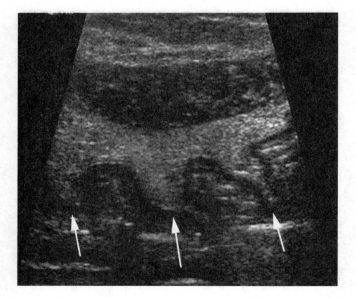

2. A 64-year-old patient presents with abdominal pain and a history of diverticulosis. What are the *arrows* in this image pointing to? Where does this pathology most commonly occur? What complications may arise?

The Kidneys

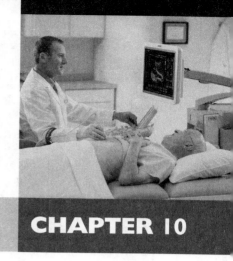

REVIEW OF GLOSSARY TERMS

Matching

Match the key terms with their definitions.

KEY TERMS

1. _____ azotemia

2. _____ BUN

3. _____ creatinine

4. _____ diuresis

5. _____ dysuria

6. _____ Gerota fascia

7. _____ hematuria

8. _____ hypernephroma

9. _____ nephrectomy

10. _____ nephropathy

11. _____ oliguria

12. _____ proteinuria

13. _____ pyuria

14. _____ urosepsis

DEFINITION

a. Blood in the urine

b. Blood test along with BUN used to measure the kidneys' ability to remove waste in the blood

c. Bacterial infection in the bloodstream as a result of a urinary tract infection

d. An overload of nitrogenous wastes such as blood urea nitrogen, uric acid, and creatinine, which occur with renal failure

e. Pus in the urine

f. Painful urination

g. Kidney disease

h. Blood test that evaluates the amount of nitrogenous waste in the blood and serves as a measure of kidney function

i. Low output of urine that is the result of many possible causes including dehydration, renal failure, or urinary obstruction

j. Increased production of urine that can occur with diabetes mellitus, acute renal failure, or increased fluid intake

k. Another term for renal cell carcinoma

l. Also known as the renal fascia; dense connective tissue that surrounds and helps anchor the kidney, adipose capsule, and the adrenal gland

m. Surgical removal of the kidney

n. Protein in the urine; sign of kidney disease

ANATOMY AND PHYSIOLOGY REVIEW

Image Labeling

Complete the labels in the images that follow.

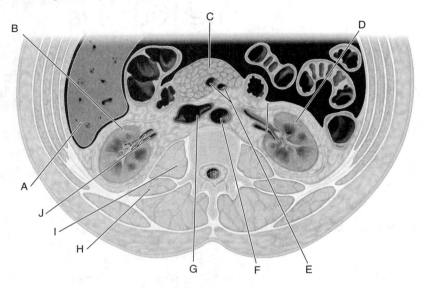

1. Retroperitoneal anatomy

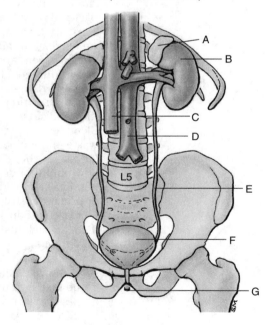

2. Urinary system

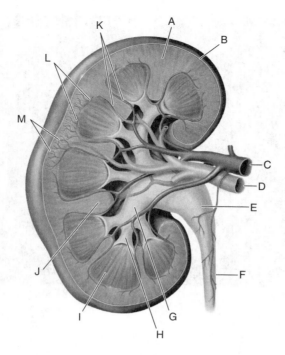

3. Renal anatomy

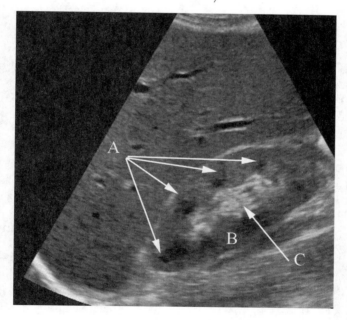

4. Renal anatomy

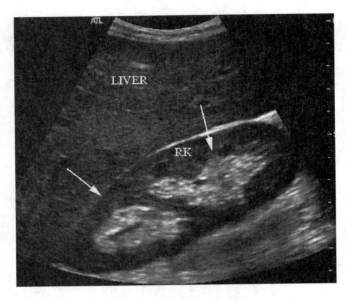

5. Congenital anomaly

CHAPTER REVIEW

Multiple Choice

Complete each question by circling the best answer.

1. Which of the following is FALSE regarding the advantage of a renal sonography examination?
   a. assess the size of the kidney, including length, width, and thickness
   b. evaluate the echogenicity of the renal cortex, medulla, and sinus
   c. evaluate the function of the kidneys
   d. differentiate between cystic and solid lesions

2. What is the functional unit of the kidney?
   a. mesonephros
   b. nephron
   c. hepatocyte
   d. pronephros

3. Approximately what gestational week do the kidneys begin to function?
   a. 4 weeks
   b. 6 weeks
   c. 8 weeks
   d. 10 weeks

4. What is the normal length of the adult kidney?
   a. 6 to 8 cm
   b. 8 to 10 cm
   c. 10 to 12 cm
   d. 12 to 14 cm

5. Which of the following surrounds the kidney and the adrenal gland and serves to anchor them to the surrounding structures?
   a. renal capsule
   b. Gerota fascia
   c. adipose capsule
   d. Glisson capsule

6. Which of the following is TRUE regarding the renal vasculature?
   a. The renal arteries arise off of the anterior aspect of the aorta.
   b. The right renal artery courses anterior to the IVC before entering the renal hilum.
   c. The left renal vein crosses posterior to the aorta before entering the IVC.
   d. Because the aorta lies to the left of midline, the right renal artery is typically longer than the left.

7. What are the extensions of cortex that lie between the renal pyramids called?
   a. columns of Bertin
   b. cortical columns
   c. fetal lobulation
   d. dromedary hump

8. What is a common renal variation in which a local bulge is seen at the lateral border of the kidney called?
   a. hypertrophied column of Bertin
   b. extrarenal pelvis
   c. fetal lobulation
   d. dromedary hump

9. What is excessive fatty infiltration of the renal pelvis called?
   a. hypertrophied column of Bertin
   b. extrarenal pelvis
   c. renal sinus lipomatosis
   d. nephrocalcinosis

10. Which of the following is NOT a laboratory test used to evaluate renal function?
    a. Blood urea nitrogen
    b. Creatinine
    c. Urinalysis
    d. Amylase

11. An RI in the adult kidney is considered normal if it is below what pulsatility index?
    a. 1
    b. 0.8
    c. 0.7
    d. 0.5

12. What is the most common congenital anomaly of the genitourinary tract?
    a. duplicated collecting system
    b. unilateral renal agenesis
    c. bilateral renal agenesis
    d. pelvic kidney

13. You are asked to evaluate a patient with a complaint of a pulsatile midline abdominal mass. Which renal condition may be responsible for this complaint?
    a. pyelonephritis
    b. pelvic kidney
    c. duplicated collecting system
    d. horseshoe kidney

14. While performing an abdominal sonography examination on a 62-year-old patient, you discover a 2-cm cystic area in the lower pole cortex. What is the most likely diagnosis?
    a. adult polycystic kidney disease
    b. simple renal cyst
    c. Von Hippel–Lindau disease
    d. medullary sponge kidney

15. Which of the following is NOT associated with adult polycystic kidney disease?
    a. bilaterally enlarged kidneys with numerous discrete cysts visible
    b. associated cysts in the liver, pancreas, and spleen
    c. small echogenic kidneys
    d. cerebral artery aneurysms located within the circle of Willis

16. What is the sonographic appearance of medullary sponge kidney?
    a. bilaterally enlarged kidneys with numerous large cysts in the region of the pyramids
    b. small, echogenic kidneys with a loss of corticomedullary junction
    c. normal-sized kidneys with echogenic cortex
    d. normal-sized kidneys with highly echogenic medullary pyramids without associated shadowing

17. What is a cyst that originates in the renal parenchyma and protrudes into the renal sinus called?
    a. simple cyst
    b. parapelvic cyst
    c. milk of calcium cyst
    d. extrarenal pelvis

18. Which of the following is NOT associated with renal cortical cysts?
    a. tuberous sclerosis
    b. von Hippel–Lindau disease
    c. adult polycystic kidney disease
    d. amyloidosis

19. Which of the following is NOT a benign tumor of the kidney?
    a. hypernephroma
    b. angiomyolipoma
    c. oncocytoma
    d. adenoma

20. If a small, well-defined, highly echogenic mass is seen in the renal cortex of a 38-year-old woman, it is most characteristic of what mass?
    a. hypernephroma
    b. oncocytoma
    c. angiomyolipoma
    d. adenoma

21. Which of the following pathologies does NOT have an increased risk of renal cell carcinoma?
    a. Von Hippel–Lindau disease
    b. medullary sponge kidney
    c. adult polycystic kidney disease
    d. tuberous sclerosis

22. A 25-year-old pregnant patient presents in her third trimester with mild right flank pain. Which of the following would you expect to find in this patient?
    a. multiple angiomyolipomas
    b. large renal cyst
    c. mild-to-moderate hydronephrosis
    d. renal cell carcinoma

23. Which of the following CANNOT cause hydronephrosis?
    a. hyperplasia of the prostate
    b. ureterocele
    c. fibroid uterus
    d. renal artery stenosis

24. What is the medical term for kidney stones?
    a. nephrolithiasis
    b. cholelithiasis
    c. nephrocalcinosis
    d. fecolithiasis

25. A patient presents with a history of medullary nephrocalcinosis. What is the typical sonographic appearance of medullary nephrocalcinosis?
    a. bilateral small echogenic kidneys
    b. enlarged kidneys with multiple distinct cystic areas
    c. normal kidney cortex with highly echogenic pyramids bilaterally
    d. bilateral hydronephrosis with thinning of the renal cortex

26. What is a common cause of acute pyelonephritis?
    a. lower urinary tract infection
    b. renal artery stenosis
    c. renal cell carcinoma
    d. colitis

27. Which of the following is FALSE regarding upper urinary tract infections?
    a. incomplete bladder emptying or stasis may lead to a UTI
    b. only respiratory infections are more common than UTIs
    c. people with diabetes or immunocompromise are more likely to have a UTI
    d. the incidence of UTIs is much higher in men

28. What is the most common cause of acute pyelonephritis?
    a. *Staphylococcus aureus*
    b. *Escherichia coli*
    c. *Pseudomonas*
    d. *Klebsiella*

29. What term describes the presence of purulent material or pus in the collecting system?
    a. hydronephrosis
    b. urosepsis
    c. pyonephrosis
    d. urolithiasis

30. A patient is referred for an abdominal sonography examination with a history of chronic medical renal disease. What is the typical sonographic appearance of this condition?
    a. bilaterally enlarged hypoechoic kidneys
    b. bilaterally enlarged kidneys with multiple discrete cysts
    c. small hypoechoic kidneys
    d. small echogenic kidneys

Fill-in-the-Blank

1. The urinary system is made up of two _____, two _____, the _____ _____, and the _____.

2. The kidneys are located in the _____ cavity.

3. During embryological development, three pairs of kidneys are formed at successive intervals: the _____, the _____, and the _____ and _____ ducts.

4. In the male, the _____ duct persists and develops into the male _____, the _____ _____, and the ejaculatory duct. In the female, the mesonephric duct develops into the _____ duct, which develops into the _____ and _____.

5. At the renal hilus, the renal _____ and renal _____, _____, nerves, and the _____ enter or exit the kidney.

6. The kidney is surrounded by three layers of supportive tissues: the innermost fibrous _____ _____, which protects against _____ and _____; the middle layer, called the _____ capsule; and the outermost layer, called _____ fascia.

7. The right kidney is _____ lower than the left due to the presence of the _____. The length of the kidneys should be within _____ cm of each other.

8. The renal _____ extends from the renal capsule to the bases of the renal _____ and the spaces between them. The renal or _____ pyramids are visualized sonographically as hypoechoic, triangular structures deep to the cortex.

9. In a normal adult, the renal cortex is _____ or _____ to the liver parenchyma. In neonates, the renal cortex is _____ or _____ to the liver parenchyma. The cortex in an adult should measure greater than _____ in thickness over the pyramids.

10. The main function of the kidneys is to remove _____ from the _____ and regulate the _____ and _____ content of the blood.

11. A urine specimen or urinalysis can be used to detect the presence of _____, _____, and _____, which could indicate _____ or _____.

12. Bilateral renal agenesis is not compatible with _____ and can be detected in utero by the absence of a _____ _____ and _____, or decreased amniotic fluid.

13. In the case of ureteral duplication, the upper pole ureter typically enters in the bladder below the trigone and may be obstructed, leading to _____ _____.

14. Complex cysts include _____ cysts, _____ cysts, and _____ or _____ cysts.

15. Calcifications in the wall of a cyst may be due to previous _____ or _____. Mural calcifications can also be associated with _____, so they may need to be evaluated by other means.

16. Milk of calcium may be found in a _____ or calyceal _____ and often forms after _____ or _____.

17. Tuberous sclerosis is a multisystemic disorder associated with bilateral renal _____ and renal _____.

18. Von Hippel–Lindau disease is an inherited disorder that can present with multiple renal _____. The cysts can contain neoplastic elements that may evolve into _____ _____ _____.

19. The most common benign kidney tumor is the _____ and is thought to be the benign counterpart of _____ _____ _____.

20. Angiomyolipomas are typically solitary and are more common in _____. _____ angiomyolipomas occur in patients with tuberous sclerosis complex.

21. Renal cell carcinoma is also known as _____ or _____, and is the most common malignant tumor of the kidney.

22. Renal cell carcinoma can spread into the perinephric _____ and renal _____. It can also spread to the _____ kidney.

23. Urothelial tumors include _____ _____ _____ and _____ _____ _____ and become clinically apparent due to painless _____.

24. Hydronephrosis is a urine _____ of the renal _____, _____ structures, and _____. Hydronephrosis makes kidneys susceptible to _____, _____ _____, and permanent _____.

25. Clinical symptoms of urolithiasis include _____ or blood in the urine, _____ if obstruction occurs, and _____ _____ as stones are passed. Stones in the right ureter may mimic symptoms of _____.

26. Trauma to the kidneys can occur during blunt or penetrating trauma. A linear absence of echoes is suggestive of a renal _____. Focal areas of hemorrhage are typically _____. A collection of blood that lies between the cortex and the renal capsule is called a _____ _____.

27. Symptoms of UTI include elevated _____ and the possibility of the presence of _____, _____, and _____ in the urine.

28. When evaluating kidneys for medical renal disease, a diffuse _____ in cortical echogenicity is typically seen. The kidneys become _____ and the medulla becomes _____.

29. _____ _____ is a leading cause of chronic renal failure and the cause of diabetic morbidity and mortality.

30. The most common cause of acute renal failure is _____ _____ _____. Renal failure is the inability of the kidneys to remove accumulated _____ from the blood. Azotemia is an overload of _____ _____, such as _____ _____ _____, _____ _____, and _____ _____ in the blood.

Short Answer

1. Common renal anatomic variants include a hypertrophied column of Bertin and an extrarenal pelvis. Describe the sonographic appearance of each of these variants and describe how you would differentiate these normal variants from a pathological condition.

2. List the main functions of the kidney. What laboratory values are used to evaluate renal function?

3. While performing a renal sonography examination, the right kidney is visualized and appears normal. The left kidney is not seen in its normal position in the left upper quadrant. What are the possible causes of this and where else would you focus your examination?

4. Renal cell carcinoma is the most common malignant tumor of the kidney. List the risk factors for developing RCC and describe what other areas should be evaluated if a renal mass is found during a sonographic examination of the abdomen.

5. List three intrinsic and three extrinsic causes of hydronephrosis. List three possible reasons for a false-positive diagnosis of hydronephrosis.

IMAGE EVALUATION/PATHOLOGY

Review the images and answer the following questions.

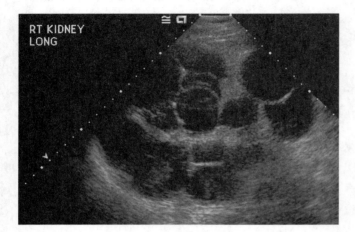

1. What pathology is seen in this image? What age does this pathology typically present? What complications may be seen with this disease?

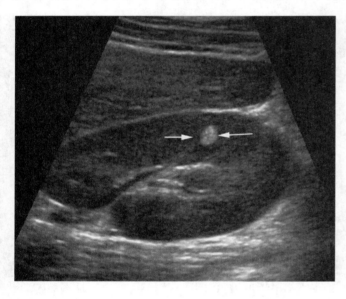

2. Describe the mass defined by the *arrows*. What is the most likely diagnosis? What disorder is associated with multiple masses of this type?

3. What condition is seen in these images? Describe the kidney seen in the images. Is this condition typically seen unilaterally or bilaterally? Are there any associated complications?

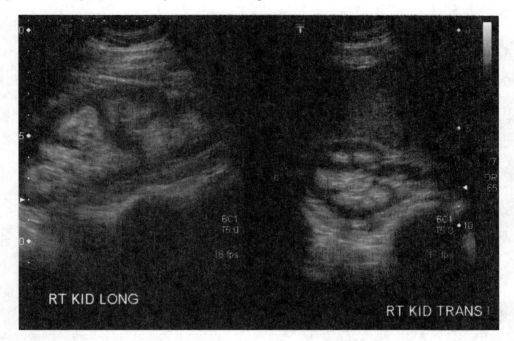

4. Describe the lesion shown in this image. What are some possible diagnoses? What further testing could be done to confirm the diagnosis?

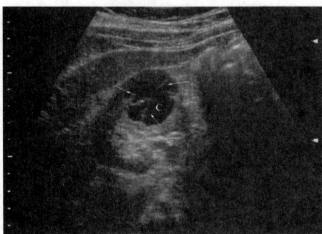

5. What pathology are the *arrows* pointing to? What symptoms are commonly associated with this pathology? How could color Doppler help with this pathology?

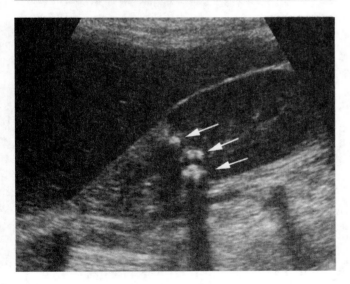

CASE STUDY

Review the images and answer the following questions.

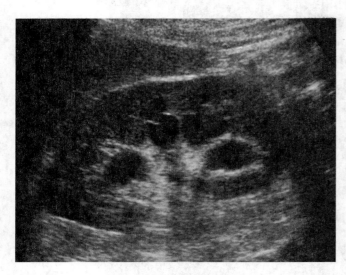

1. A 42-year-old man presents with severe right flank pain and hematuria. He has a history of bilateral kidney stones. What is seen in this image of the right kidney? If a kidney stone is causing an obstruction at the right ureteropelvic junction, what structure(s) will be dilated? What if the stone is at the right ureterovesical junction?

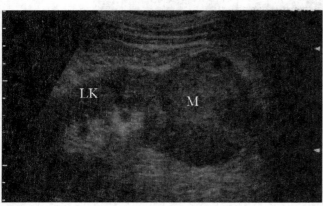

2. A 58-year-old man presents with gross hematuria and mild left flank discomfort. Describe what is seen in this image. What is the most likely diagnosis? Describe other possible sonographic appearances of this pathology.

The Lower Urinary System

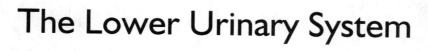
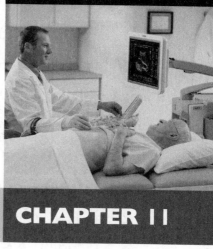

REVIEW OF GLOSSARY TERMS

Matching

Match the key terms with their definitions.

KEY TERMS

1. _____ cystitis

2. _____ cystoscopy

3. _____ exstrophy

4. _____ hematuria

5. _____ diverticula

6. _____ trabeculated bladder

7. _____ VCUG

DEFINITIONS

a. Presence of red blood cells in the urine
b. Out-pouching of the bladder wall
c. Procedure in which a scope is used to evaluate the urethra, bladder, and pelvic ureters
d. Irregular bladder wall frequently seen in patients with longstanding obstruction or neurogenic bladder
e. Fluoroscopic exam used to evaluate for urinary reflux
f. Congenital anomaly in which part of the urinary bladder is located outside the abdominal wall
g. Inflammation of the urinary bladder

ANATOMY AND PHYSIOLOGY REVIEW

Image Labeling

Complete the labels in the images that follow.

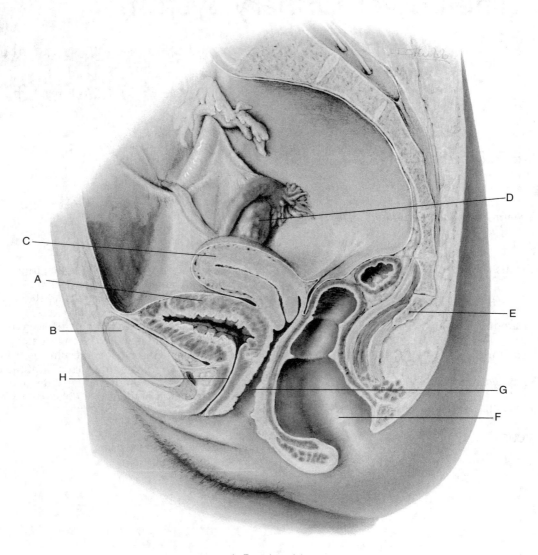

1. Female pelvis

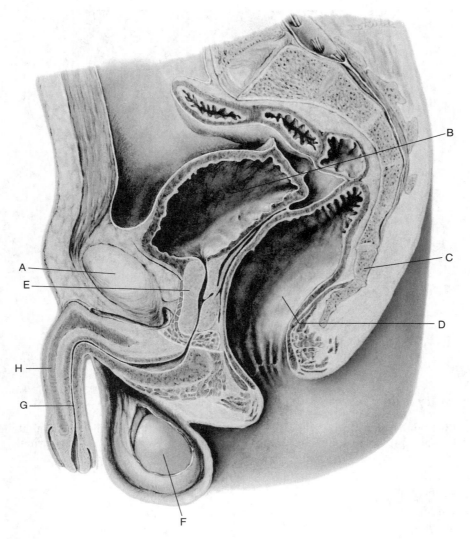

2. Male pelvis

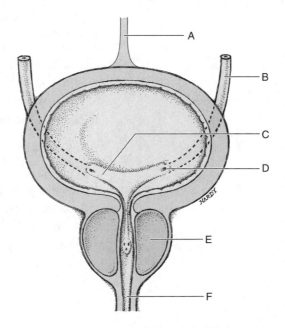

3. Lateral view of the male pelvis

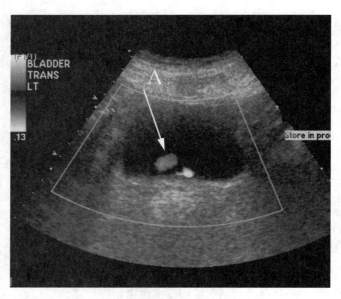

4. Color Doppler of the urinary bladder

CHAPTER REVIEW

Multiple Choice

Complete each question by circling the best answer.

1. The bladder is lined with a mucous membrane. What tissue that allows for expansion makes up this membrane?
   a. squamous epithelium
   b. transitional epithelium
   c. intimal epithelium
   d. urogenital epithelium

2. Which of the following statements regarding the urethra is FALSE?
   a. The female urethra is 3 to 4 cm long and transports urine from the body.
   b. The male urethra is longer than the female urethra and has a dual function.
   c. The internal urethral sphincter is formed by a thickening of the detrusor muscle.
   d. The external urethral sphincter is formed of skeletal muscle and is under involuntary control.

3. What term describes the involuntary emptying of the bladder?
   a. micturition
   b. incontinence
   c. retention
   d. voiding

4. What term describes the inability to empty the bladder even when it is full of urine?
   a. micturition
   b. incontinence
   c. retention
   d. voiding

5. While evaluating the urinary bladder in a patient with a history of lower urinary tract infection, you suspect the bladder wall may be thickened. What is the normal measurement of the bladder wall when the bladder is distended?
   a. less than 7 mm
   b. less than 5 mm
   c. less than 3 mm
   d. less than 2 mm

6. A 26-year-old woman presents with dysuria, fever, and pelvic pain. The bladder wall is diffusely thickened and hypoechoic. The kidneys appear normal. What is the most likely cause of these findings?
   a. bladder neoplasm
   b. bladder outlet obstruction
   c. cystitis
   d. ureterocele

7. While evaluating the bladder with color Doppler, you visualize ureteral jets on the left side but are unable to detect a jet on the right. What might this indicate?

   a. hydronephrosis

   b. urinary tract infection

   c. bladder outlet obstruction

   d. ureteral obstruction

8. Which of the following statements regarding bladder diverticula is FALSE?

   a. A bladder diverticula will always empty completely with voiding.

   b. A diverticula may be the result of a chronic bladder obstruction.

   c. Stones or tumor may occur in a bladder diverticula.

   d. A large bladder diverticula may mimic an ovarian cyst.

9. You receive a request to evaluate the urinary system in a male newborn with suspected bladder outlet obstruction. What is the most common cause of bladder outlet obstruction?

   a. bilateral renal agenesis

   b. ectopic ureterocele

   c. vesicoureteral reflux

   d. posterior urethral valves

10. Which of the following CANNOT cause bladder outlet obstruction?

    a. congenital urethral stricture

    b. stone at the ureteropelvic junction

    c. ureterocele

    d. posterior urethral valves

11. What is a condition in which the bladder is herniated through a defect in the anterior abdominal wall called?

    a. bladder exstrophy

    b. complete duplication of the bladder

    c. bladder diverticula

    d. ureterocele

12. A female infant presents with a low-grade fever and palpable abdominal mass just superior to the urinary bladder. Sonographically, a cystic mass is seen in this area. A connection to the bladder cannot be identified. What does this structure likely represent?

    a. duplicated bladder

    b. bladder diverticula

    c. ureterocele

    d. urachal cyst

13. You are performing an examination of the urinary tract on a male infant with a history of urinary tract infections. You visualize a round cystic structure within the bladder lumen. With color Doppler you are able to detect a consistent ureteral jet coming from the area. What is the most likely diagnosis?

    a. Foley catheter in the bladder

    b. bladder diverticula

    c. ureterocele

    d. bladder mass

14. A patient presents with a history of lower urinary tract infections. The bladder wall appears normal; however, a small echogenic area is seen along the posterior wall of the bladder. Acoustic shadowing is present posterior to the area and the echogenic foci moves with a change in patient position. What does this echogenic foci represent?

    a. a bladder calculi

    b. a calcified bladder mass

    c. Foley catheter in the urinary bladder

    d. ectopic ureterocele

15. Which of the following statements regarding reflux is FALSE?

    a. The vesicoureteral junction normally protects the kidney from the backflow of infected urine.

    b. The vesicoureteral junction normally allows the flow of urine both into and out of the bladder.

    c. High-pressure reflux is a major cause of chronic renal failure.

    d. When reflux is in process, dilation of the ureter may be seen with sonography.

16. The ureterovesical junction describes what anatomic location?

    a. Proximal ureter joins the renal pelvis.

    b. Distal ureter joins the urinary bladder.

    c. Distal urethra joins the urinary bladder.

    d. Proximal urethra joins the urinary bladder.

17. A patient presents with a history of right ureterovesical junction obstruction. Which of the following would NOT be an expected finding?

    a. right megaureter

    b. right-sided hydronephrosis

    c. ectopic ureterocele

    d. left-sided hydronephrosis

18. On sonographic examination, your patient is noted to have a thickened bladder wall. Which of the following CANNOT cause bladder wall thickening?

    a. bladder outlet obstruction

    b. neurogenic bladder

    c. overhydration

    d. cystitis

19. What term describes a fluid collection that occurs as a result of bladder trauma?
    a. urinoma
    b. lymphocele
    c. ureterocele
    d. diverticula

20. What is the most common type of bladder malignancy?
    a. adenocarcinoma
    b. squamous cell carcinoma
    c. lymphoma
    d. transitional cell carcinoma

Fill-in-the-Blank

1. The lower urinary tract consists of the pelvic _____, _____, and _____.

2. Initially, the bladder is contiguous with the _____, which eventually becomes the _____, which extends from the apex of the bladder to the _____.

3. The bladder wall is composed of four layers: the innermost transitional epithelium, the _____, the muscle layer, which is called the _____ muscle, and the fibrous _____.

4. The ureters are constricted in three places: at the _____ junction, as they cross the _____ vessels, and at the _____ junction.

5. The _____ is the terminal portion of the urinary tract. The _____ _____ _____ is an _____ muscle that keeps the urethra closed and prevents leaking. Contraction _____ this sphincter, and _____ closes it.

6. The thickness of the bladder wall should measure less than _____ when it is distended and less than _____ when empty or partially distended.

7. On transverse sections, the shape of the bladder superiorly is _____, whereas more inferiorly, the shape is _____. On longitudinal sections, the bladder shape is more _____.

8. If the ureters are dilated, they can be visualized as round structures _____ to the urinary bladder in the _____ plane.

9. Bladder volume is calculated using the formula for an _____. The formula is _____ × _____ × _____ × _____.

10. _____ or _____ scanning techniques may be used to evaluate the female urethra. _____, or small defects in the urethral wall, may be identified.

11. A posterior urethral valve is a mucosal flap originating from the _____ that obstructs urine flow and causes bladder _____ _____. Sonographically, the _____ urethra is elongated and dilated. The bladder wall is typically _____.

12. An _____ ureter does not insert into the typical location in the bladder trigone. This ureter typically arises from the _____ pelvis of a _____ kidney and inserts _____ and more _____ toward the bladder base.

13. A _____ is a cyst-like enlargement of the lower end of the ureter. If the ureteral opening is narrowed, _____ and _____ may be present. If the ureterocele obstructs the opening to the urethra, _____ _____ _____ may occur.

14. If the _____ fails to close properly, an open channel between the bladder and umbilicus may form. Complications include _____, _____, or _____ formation.

15. Inflammation of the bladder is called _____. This infection is typically caused by the bacteria _____ _____. If the infection travels to the kidneys, it can cause _____.

16. Predisposing factors to bladder stone formation include increased _____ of salts in the urine, _____ of the urinary tract, and urinary tract _____ or _____.

17. A patient with a _____ bladder has lost voluntary control of voiding due to a disturbance somewhere along the neural pathway. The bladder may be either _____ or _____, depending on the nature of the damage.

18. During a cesarean section, a potential space is created between the bladder and the uterus known as a _____ _____. A _____ can form in this potential space following surgery. A fever and leukocytosis can indicate that this area has become _____.

19. The most common symptom of a bladder neoplasm is _____ _____. Sonography typically displays _____ wall thickening. Metastatic bladder tumors may occur by direct extension from primary tumors of the _____, _____, _____, and _____.

20. Any condition that causes urinary stasis or obstruction predisposes a patient to _____ formation and _____.

Short Answer

1. Describe two possible patient preparations used for a transabdominal sonographic evaluation of the urinary bladder. What other methods besides the transabdominal approach are used to evaluate the lower urinary tract?

2. What role does color Doppler play in the evaluation of the urinary bladder? Discuss three examples.

3. What is an ectopic ureterocele? How does this pathology cause hydronephrosis? Describe the sonographic appearance of this pathology.

4. What mechanism is in place to protect the kidneys from infected urine in the bladder? What problems can occur when this mechanism malfunctions?

5. Describe the sonographic appearance of a neurogenic bladder. What causes these changes?

IMAGE EVALUATION/PATHOLOGY

Review the images and answer the following questions.

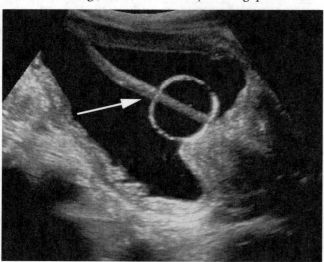

1. What structure is the *arrow* pointing to?

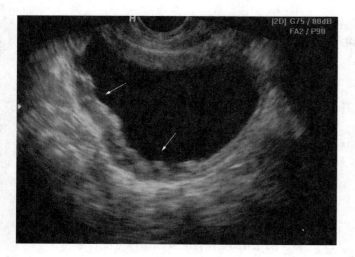

2. What are the *arrows* pointing to? Does this structure appear normal? What can cause thickening of the bladder wall?

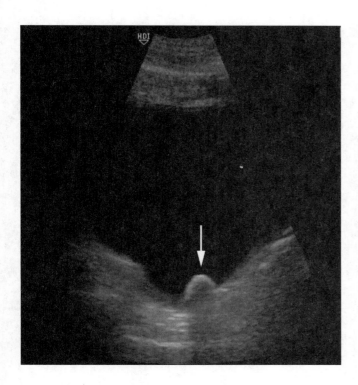

3. What is the *arrow* pointing to in this image? List two predisposing factors for this pathology. What complications may occur?

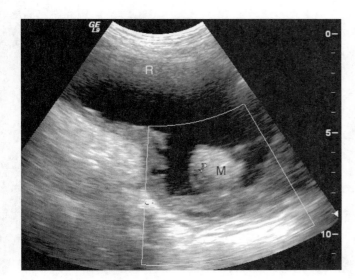

4. Describe what is seen in this image. What is the likely diagnosis? What could mimic this pathology?

CASE STUDY

Review the image and answer the following questions.

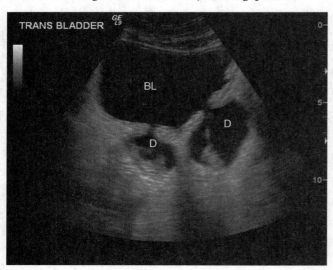

1. A 26-year-old woman presents with a recent history of a lower urinary tract infection with symptoms of urinary frequency and dysuria. What do you see in this image? How does this pathology predispose the patient to urinary tract infections?

The Prostate Gland

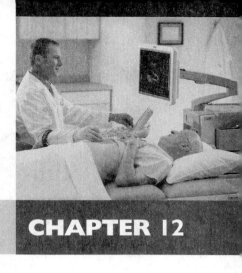

REVIEW OF GLOSSARY TERMS

Matching

Match the key terms with their definitions.

KEY TERMS

1. _____ apex

2. _____ base

3. _____ corpora amylacea

4. _____ Eiffel Tower sign

5. _____ ejaculatory ducts

6. _____ endogenous calculi

7. _____ exogenous calculi

8. _____ seminal vesicles

9. _____ surgical capsule

10. _____ vas deferens

11. _____ verumontanum

DEFINITIONS

a. Reproductive duct that extends from the epididymis to the ejaculatory duct

b. Superior portion of the prostate gland, which is located below the inferior margin of the urinary bladder

c. Calculi found within the urethra

d. Calcifications commonly seen in the inner gland of the prostate

e. Inferior portion of the prostate gland, which is located superior to the urogenital diaphragm

f. A longitudinal ridge within the prostatic urethral wall where the orifices of the ejaculatory ducts are located on either side

g. Calculi formation within the substance of the prostate

h. Shadowing created by calcification in the area of the urethra and verumontanum

i. A pair of tubular glands which extend from outpouching of the vas deferens

j. Demarcation between the inner gland and the outer gland, which normally appears hypoechoic

k. Duct that passes through the central zone and empties into the urethra; originates from the combination of the vas deferens and the seminal vesicle

ANATOMY AND PHYSIOLOGY REVIEW

Image Labeling

Complete the labels in the images that follow.

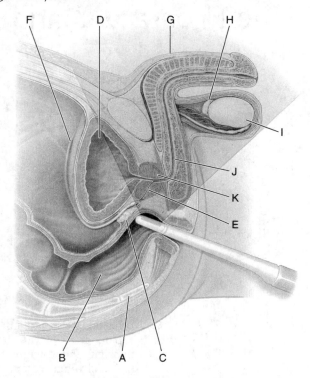

1. Male pelvis

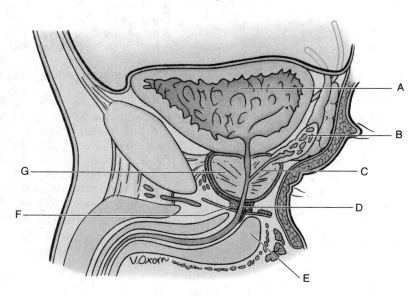

2. Sagittal view of the male pelvis

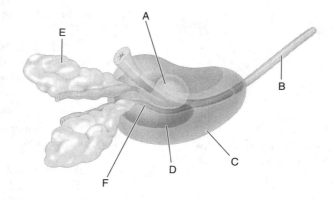

3. Zonal anatomy

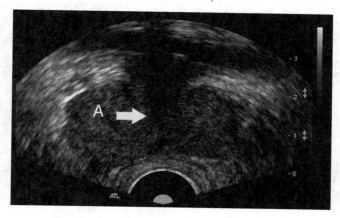

4. Normal prostate anatomy

CHAPTER REVIEW

Multiple Choice

Complete each question by circling the best answer.

1. Which structure travels within the central zone of the prostate gland and joins the urethra?
   a. ejaculatory duct
   b. seminal vesicle
   c. vas deferens
   d. verumontanum

2. Which of the following is NOT a zone within the glandular tissue of the prostate gland?
   a. peripheral zone
   b. epithelial zone
   c. central zone
   d. periurethral zone

3. Which of the glandular zones of the prostate is the largest?
   a. peripheral zone
   b. periurethral zone
   c. central zone
   d. transition zone

4. In which zone does prostate cancer and prostatitis most often occur?
   a. peripheral zone
   b. periurethral zone
   c. central zone
   d. transition zone

5. Your patient presents for a sonography examination to evaluate for benign prostatic hypertrophy. Which zone is most affected by BPH?
   a. peripheral zone
   b. periurethral zone
   c. central zone
   d. transition zone

6. Which blood test is used to identify men at increased risk of prostate cancer?
   a. AFP
   b. CA-125
   c. PSA
   d. AST

7. The apex of the prostate is located inferior to the verumontanum and is made up predominantly of which zone?
   a. peripheral zone
   b. periurethral zone
   c. central zone
   d. transition zone

8. The base of the prostate is located superior to the verumontanum and is made up predominantly of which zone?
   a. peripheral zone
   b. periurethral zone
   c. central zone
   d. transition zone

9. Which of the following cysts is associated with genital anomalies such as hypospadias?
   a. Müllerian duct cyst
   b. utricle cyst
   c. seminal vesicle cyst
   d. prostatic cyst

10. Which of the following cysts will contain spermatozoa?
    a. Müllerian duct cyst
    b. utricle cyst
    c. seminal vesicle cyst
    d. prostatic cyst

11. A diabetic patient presents with fever, urinary frequency, low back pain, and hematuria. While scanning the prostate the gland, you notice a focal complex area that has increased blood flow. What is the most likely diagnosis given the patient's history?
    a. BPH
    b. prostate cancer
    c. prostatic cyst
    d. prostatic abscess

12. What is the most common symptomatic condition to affect the prostate gland?
    a. BPH
    b. prostate cancer
    c. prostatic cyst
    d. prostatitis

13. Your patient states that he has had a transurethral resection or TURP procedure. What condition does this procedure treat?
    a. prostate cancer
    b. prostatic abscess
    c. prostatitis
    d. BPH

14. Which of the following statements regarding BPH is FALSE?
    a. BPH is commonly seen in men over the age of 40 with a peak incidence around 60.
    b. BPH causes the prostate to appear more rounded than normal.
    c. BPH affects the central zone of the prostate.
    d. BPH causes urinary symptoms of frequency, nocturia, and difficulty starting a stream.

15. What is the sonographic appearance of the prostate gland in patients with benign prostatic hypertrophy?
    a. hypoechoic
    b. hyperechoic
    c. heterogeneous
    d. the appearance of BPH could include all of the above

16. Where does corpora amylacea occur most often?
    a. superior segment of the prostate
    b. inferior segment of the prostate
    c. posterior segment of the prostate
    d. anterior segment of the prostate

17. Patients with prostate cancer may present with which of the following symptoms?
    a. an abnormal PSA level
    b. an abnormal DRE
    c. bladder outlet obstruction
    d. patients may present with all of the above symptoms

18. A definitive diagnosis of prostate cancer can be made by which of the following procedures?
    a. DRE
    b. TRUS
    c. ultrasound-guided biopsy
    d. PSA level

19. What is the predictive value of TRUS alone for diagnosing prostate cancer diagnosis?
    a. less than 10 percent
    b. 25 percent
    c. 50 percent
    d. 75 percent

20. Which of the following statements regarding ultrasound-guided prostate biopsy is TRUE?
    a. Prostate biopsy is only performed if a discrete lesion can be identified with ultrasound.
    b. The method of choice is the transperineal approach.
    c. Prostate biopsy is commonly done at known sites of anatomic weakness.
    d. Prostate biopsy is routinely done from a transabdominal approach with a full urinary bladder.

Fill-in-the-Blank

1. TRUS is an acronym for _____ _____.

2. TRUS of the prostate can be used to evaluate the prostate in cases of _____, _____, _____ _____ _____ _____, and _____ abnormalities. It can also be used to guide _____ and treatment procedures.

3. The _____ ducts are responsible for development of the male reproductive system, whereas the _____ form the female reproductive system.

4. The prostate is shaped like a _____ and measures _____ on average.

5. The cephalic portion of the gland is the _____, whereas the caudal portion is the _____. The _____ travels through the center of the prostate gland.

6. Sonographically, the peripheral zone tissue is _____ and _____. The _____ _____ separates the peripheral zone from the central zone. The echogenicity of the central zone is _____ than the peripheral zone.

7. Sonographic characteristics of prostate disease include changes in _____, _____ of the gland, and a distorted _____.

8. When performing an examination of the prostate, the image is typically _____ with the near field at the _____ of the image and the far field at the _____ of the image. In the transverse plane, the right lobe of the gland is at the _____ side of the image and the left lobe of the gland is on the _____ side of the image.

9. The capsule of the prostate gland should appear _____ and without _____.

10. The most common of the pelvic cystic masses are the _____ duct and _____ cysts.

11. A utricle cyst is _____ in origin and is typically associated with genital anomalies such as _____, _____ testicles, and _____ anomalies.

12. The majority of patients with seminal vesicle cyst also have ipsilateral _____ _____.

13. The most common cysts are typically the result of BPH and are seen in the _____ zone of the prostate.

14. Prostatic calculi are divided into _____ calculi and _____ calculi. _____ calculi are found within the prostate gland and form from _____ fluid. _____ calculi are found within the urethra and are derived from _____.

15. _____ calculi can produce what is known as the "Eiffel Tower" appearance.

16. Patients with acute bacterial prostatitis present with a _____, along with _____ _____ and _____ pain. Large numbers of _____ _____ will be present within the urine.

17. The prostate is infected by organisms ascending from the _____ _____. There is a greater incidence of prostatitis within the _____ zone.

18. The most common sonographic finding in patients with a history of prostatitis is a _____ _____ in the periurethral area. The peripheral zone may also have a _____ echo pattern.

19. The most common cancer in American men is _____ _____. The majority are diagnosed in men over the age of _____.

20. The most common type of prostate cancer is _____ and occurs most commonly in the _____ zone. Most are _____, as opposed to solitary lesions.

Short Answer

1. What are the most common indications for sonography of the prostate? Is TRUS of the prostate typically used for screening purposes?

2. Describe the sonographic technique used to evaluate the prostate gland, including patient preparation, positioning, image orientation, and any contraindications to the study.

3. Calcifications are commonly seen in the prostate gland. What conditions can cause calcifications within the prostate?

4. Prostate cancer is the second most deadly male cancer, making its diagnosis an important one. Describe the sonographic appearance of prostate cancer. Is ultrasound a good screening tool for prostate cancer? Why or why not?

5. Describe the method most commonly used for ultrasound-guided prostate biopsy, including patient preparation and technique.

IMAGE EVALUATION/PATHOLOGY

Review the images and answer the following questions.

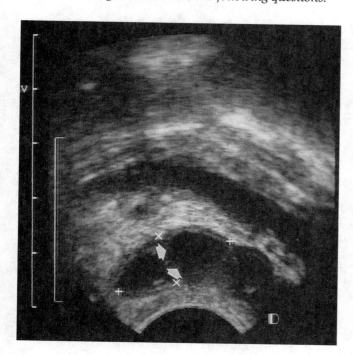

1. This image was taken lateral to the base of the prostate. What structure is imaged here? Does this structure appear normal? If not, what could cause this?

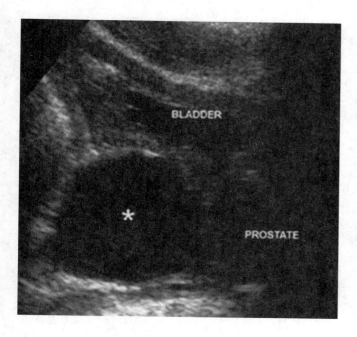

2. A cystic structure is demonstrated in this male pelvis between the bladder and the rectum. What is the likely diagnosis? What type of symptoms might the patient experience?

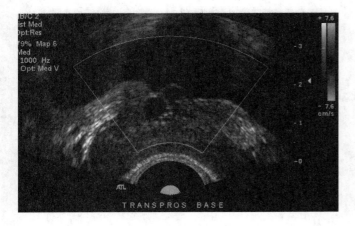

3. This image demonstrates cystic structures in the base of the prostate gland in an asymptomatic patient. What is a possible diagnosis?

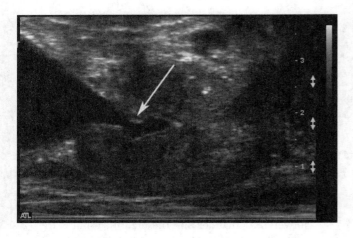

4. This 55-year-old patient has a history of severe BPH. What could cause the changes seen in the center of this prostate gland? How does this work?

CASE STUDY

Review the image and answer the following questions.

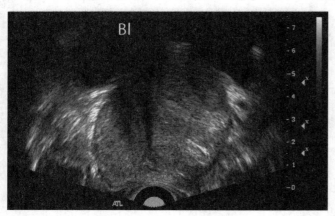

1. A 54-year-old patient presents with symptoms of urinary frequency and nocturia. What is seen in this image of the prostate gland? In what age range does this typically occur? Which zone is typically affected?

The Adrenal Glands

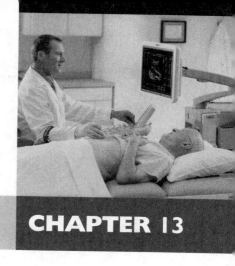

CHAPTER 13

REVIEW OF GLOSSARY TERMS

Matching

Match the terms with their definitions.

KEY TERMS

1. _____ ACTH

2. _____ adrenal cortex

3. _____ adrenal medulla

4. _____ endoscopic ultrasound

5. _____ MEN

DEFINITIONS

a. An ultrasound transducer that is inserted in the mouth or anus to visualize the walls of the digestive tract and surrounding organs

b. Inner portion of the adrenal gland that secretes the catecholamines epinephrine and norepinephrine

c. A group of autosomal dominant disorders characterized by benign and malignant tumors of the endocrine glands

d. Hormone secreted by the pituitary gland that causes the adrenal gland to produce and release corticosteroids

e. Outer parenchyma of the adrenal gland that secretes corticoids, including cortisol and aldosterone

ANATOMY AND PHYSIOLOGY REVIEW

Image Labeling

Complete the labels in the images that follow.

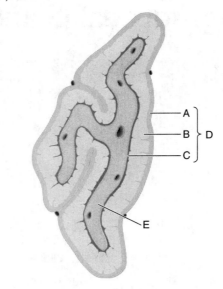

1. Adrenal anatomy

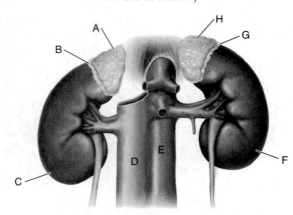

2. Retroperitoneal anatomy

RIGHT

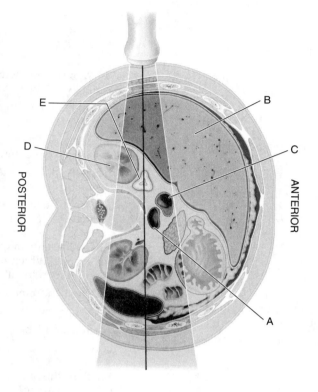

LEFT

3. Right scan plane

LEFT

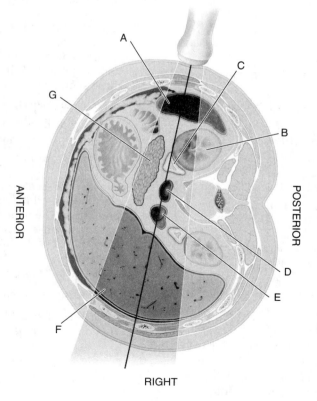

RIGHT

4. Left scan plane

CHAPTER REVIEW

Multiple Choice

Complete each question by circling the best answer.

1. The adrenal gland is really two glands in one organ. What is the adrenal gland composed of?
   a. two endocrine glands
   b. two exocrine glands
   c. one exocrine gland and one endocrine gland
   d. none of the above

2. Which of the following is NOT one of the adrenal cortex zones?
   a. zona glomerulosa
   b. zona fasciculata
   c. zona muscularis
   d. zona reticularis

3. Which of the following regarding the anatomy of the adrenal glands is FALSE?
   a. The right adrenal gland lies posterior and lateral to the IVC.
   b. The right adrenal gland has a triangular shape.
   c. The right adrenal gland is larger than the left.
   d. The left adrenal gland has a crescent or semilunar shape.

4. Which of the following is NOT a cortical hormone?
   a. cortisol
   b. adrenalin
   c. androgen
   d. estrogen

5. Which of the following statements regarding the medulla is FALSE?
   a. The medulla synthesizes epinephrine and norepinephrine.
   b. Release of the hormones is stimulated through the sympathetic nervous system.
   c. The medullary hormones are essential to life and must be replaced if the adrenal glands are removed.
   d. The anticipation of stress or pain causes the release of the medullary hormones.

6. Which of the following statements regarding sonography evaluation of the adrenal gland is FALSE?
   a. The liver can frequently be used as an acoustic window when evaluating the right adrenal gland.
   b. The right adrenal gland can be visualized posterior to the crus of the diaphragm.
   c. The left adrenal gland can be visualized between the left kidney and the aorta.
   d. The left adrenal gland may be imaged with the patient in the cava-suprarenal line position.

7. Which of the following statements regarding adrenal pathology is TRUE?
   a. A right-sided adrenal mass may displace the kidney anteriorly.
   b. A left-sided adrenal mass may displace the splenic vein anteriorly.
   c. A left-sided adrenal mass may displace the kidney superiorly.
   d. A right-sided adrenal mass may displace the right renal vein posteriorly.

8. In hypoadrenalism, patients have a decreased steroid output. Which of the following conditions is a form of hypoadrenalism?
   a. Conn syndrome
   b. Cushing syndrome
   c. aldosteronism
   d. Addison disease

9. Which of the following is NOT a form of hyperadrenalism?
   a. Conn syndrome
   b. Cushing syndrome
   c. aldosteronism
   d. Addison disease

10. A patient presents with elevated serum glucose levels, hyperpigmentation of the skin, and thinning of the abdominal tissue with red striations seen on the abdominal wall. Which of the following could cause these symptoms?
    a. Addison disease
    b. Cushing syndrome
    c. Pheochromocytoma
    d. Conn syndrome

11. A patient presents with hyperpigmentation of the skin, decreased kidney function, fatigue, and hypotension. The patient also complains of gastrointestinal concerns such as diarrhea and weight loss. Which of the following could cause these symptoms?
    a. Addison disease
    b. Cushing syndrome
    c. pheochromocytoma
    d. Conn syndrome

12. What is the most common cause of Cushing syndrome?
    a. long-term use of insulin
    b. tuberculosis infection
    c. alcoholism
    d. long-term use of steroids such as prednisone

13. What is the most common cause of Conn syndrome?
    a. long-term use of steroids such as prednisone
    b. tuberculosis infection
    c. aldosterone-producing adrenal adenoma
    d. pheochromocytoma

14. What are the principle clinical symptoms of Conn syndrome?
    a. diabetes
    b. hypernatremia and hypokalemia
    c. hypertension and headaches
    d. hypercalcemia and hypovolemia

15. Which of the following is common in a patient who presents with a history of highly elevated blood pressure, headache, and rapid heartbeat?
    a. Conn syndrome
    b. Cushing syndrome
    c. pheochromocytoma
    d. cortical adenoma

16. Which of the following tumors occurs in the adrenal medulla?
    a. adenoma
    b. pheochromocytoma
    c. myelolipoma
    d. adenocarcinoma

17. Which of the following describes the most common appearance of the adrenal adenoma?
    a. small, round, homogeneous hypoechoic lesions
    b. large hyperechoic lesion with irregular borders
    c. complex lesion of varying size with increased through transmission
    d. small hypoechoic lesion with a calcified rim

18. Which of the following may be seen in patients with MEN syndrome?
    a. acute hypoadrenalism
    b. primary adrenal insufficiency
    c. adrenal myelolipoma
    d. cortical adenoma

19. A patient presents for an abdominal sonography examination to rule out a pheochromocytoma. Which of the following increases a person's risk of developing a pheochromocytoma?
    a. MEN syndrome
    b. Addison disease
    c. cortical adenoma
    d. neuroblastoma

20. Which of the following statements regarding pheochromocytoma is FALSE?
    a. All pheochromocytomas are malignant.
    b. Pheochromocytomas may be unilateral or bilateral.
    c. Pheochromocytomas occur more frequently in patients with hereditary endocrine tumor syndromes.
    d. Patients with a pheochromocytoma have elevated levels of urinary catecholamines.

Fill-in-the-Blank

1. Transabdominal as well as _____ and _____ approaches can be used to evaluate the adrenal glands.

2. The adrenal gland is made up of the _____ and the _____ and is combined within a common _____.

3. Initially, the fetal adrenal gland is _____ than the kidney.

4. The adrenal glands lie _____, _____, and _____ to the kidneys.

5. _____ _____ fascia surrounds both the kidney and adrenal gland. _____ tissue also surrounds each gland and separates it from the kidney.

6. The adrenal cortex makes up _____ percent of the gland. The cortical hormones are _____, _____, and _____.

7. Hormone secretion in the adrenal gland is controlled by a _____ _____ mechanism. _____ blood levels of hormones trigger the hypothalamus to secrete _____, which triggers the pituitary to release _____, which works to increase adrenal hormone activity.

8. The medulla secretes _____ hormones, similar to the _____ and _____ _____ glands. Hormones are produced in the _____ or _____ cells.

9. The adult adrenal glands are _____ cm long, _____ cm wide, and _____ mm thick.

10. The right adrenal gland is seen _____ to the kidney and _____ to the right crus of the diaphragm. The left adrenal gland is _____ to the left crus of the diaphragm and _____ or _____ to the aorta.

11. With right adrenal gland disease, the _____ _____ _____, _____, and _____ _____ _____ may be displaced anteriorly, while the right kidney is displaced _____ or _____.

12. An enlarged left adrenal gland may displace the splenic vein _____ and the left kidney _____ or _____.

13. Adrenal hemorrhage is most common in _____ after a difficult delivery. _____ are common with resolving hematoma and may shadow.

14. Chronic primary hypoadrenalism, or _____ disease, causes an increase in the pituitary's production of _____, which causes changes in _____ color.

15. Acute hypoadrenalism, or _____ _____ _____, occurs due to widespread _____, _____, or _____ _____ septicemia.

16. The term for an unexpected mass found during an imaging procedure is _____. In patients without a history of cancer, the majority of these masses were _____, whereas in patients with a history of cancer the majority of the masses were found to be _____.

17. Adrenal adenomas may be part of the _____ syndrome. They may be _____, and in that case may cause _____ syndrome.

18. Adenocarcinomas often produce _____. The tumors are typically large and may show anechoic zones of _____ and _____. Cortical cancers may invade the _____ vein, _____, and _____.

19. Patients with pheochromocytoma typically present with _____, _____, _____, and _____. Symptoms result from an increased _____ secretion.

20. The adrenal gland is the _____ most common site for metastases. Metastases tend to be _____. The masses may indent the posterior wall of the _____ and displace the kidneys _____.

Short Answer

1. CT is the imaging modality of choice for primary imaging of the adrenal glands, although sonography can also play a role. In what instances would sonography be used instead of CT? List four indications for sonography of the adrenal glands.

2. Chronic primary hypoadrenalism, or Addison disease, results in insufficient secretion of the adrenocortical hormones. What causes Addison disease and what are the common symptoms?

3. What causes Cushing syndrome? What are the common clinical symptoms of Cushing syndrome?

4. What is an incidentaloma? What might an adrenal incidentaloma represent?

IMAGE EVALUATION/PATHOLOGY

Review the images and answer the following questions.

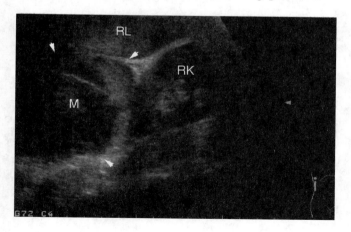

1. The mass (*M*) seen in this sagittal image represents an adrenal hemorrhage. Where is the mass located in relationship to the right kidney? What helps distinguish this extrarenal mass from a renal mass?

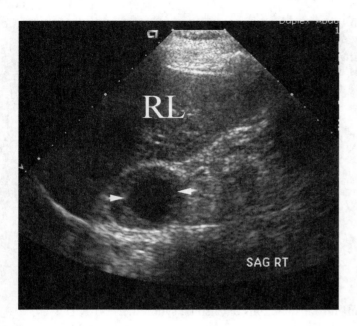

2. Describe the lesion located between the *arrows* in this image. What symptoms would you expect from this type of lesion?

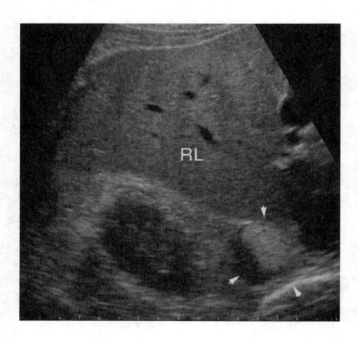

3. Describe the mass indicated by the *arrows* in this transverse image. Describe the location of the mass in reference to the right kidney. What is the most likely diagnosis?

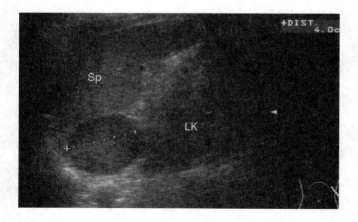

4. Describe the mass seen between the calipers in this image. This mass was diagnosed as an adenoma. Are adrenal adenomas typically symptomatic and, if so, what symptoms do they cause?

CASE STUDY

Review the images and answer the following questions.

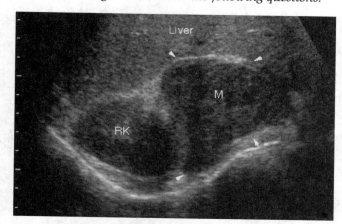

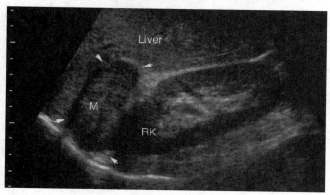

1. A 57-year-old patient with a history of lung cancer presents for an abdominal sonography examination. Describe the mass seen in these images. How is the mass distinguished from a liver or renal mass? Where is the mass located in relation to the right kidney? Where else in the abdomen would you focus your examination after identifying this mass?

The Retroperitoneum

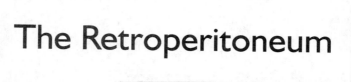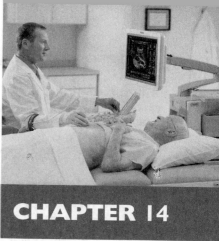

CHAPTER 14

REVIEW OF GLOSSARY TERMS

Matching

Match the terms with their definitions.

KEY TERMS

1. _____ abscess

2. _____ adenopathy

3. _____ extravasate

4. _____ fascia

5. _____ great vessels

6. _____ hematoma

7. _____ HIV

8. _____ mass effect

9. _____ metastasis

10. _____ orthogonal

11. _____ primary neoplasm

12. _____ urinoma

DEFINITION

a. Distortion or displacement of normal anatomy due to a mass, neoplasm, or fluid collection

b. Fluid such as blood, bile, or urine that is forced out or leaks out of its normal vessel into the surrounding tissues or potential spaces

c. A thin, sheet-like tissue that separates muscles

d. A pocket of infection typically containing pus, blood, and degenerating tissue

e. Planes that are perpendicular, or 90 degrees, to each other

f. The spread of cancer from the site at which it first arose to a distant site

g. Enlargement of lymph nodes due to inflammation, primary neoplasia, or metastasis

h. A term used to describe the aorta and IVC together

i. An extravasated urine collection due to a tear of the urinary collecting system

j. An extravasated collection of blood localized within a potential space or tissues

k. A new growth of benign or malignant origin

l. A blood-borne virus that attacks T-lymphocytes, resulting in their destruction or impairment, eventually leading to AIDS

ANATOMY AND PHYSIOLOGY REVIEW

Image Labeling

Complete the labels in the images that follow.

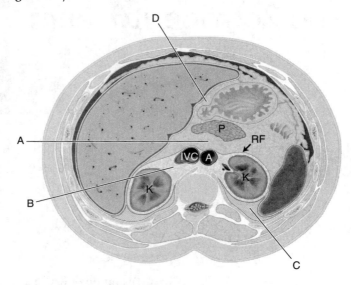

1. Retroperitoneal compartments

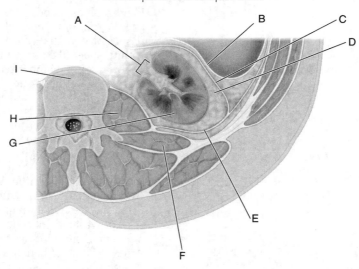

2. Retroperitoneum

CHAPTER REVIEW

Multiple Choice

Complete each question by circling the best answer.

1. Which of the following is NOT a retroperitoneal compartment?
   a. anterior pararenal space
   b. perirenal space
   c. posterior parietal space
   d. posterior pararenal space

2. Which retroperitoneal space contains no organs?
   a. anterior pararenal space
   b. perirenal space
   c. posterior parietal space
   d. posterior pararenal space

3. Which of the following is NOT found within the anterior pararenal space?
   a. pancreas
   b. adrenal glands
   c. ascending colon
   d. distal CBD

4. Which of the following is NOT found within the perirenal space?
   a. kidneys
   b. great vessels
   c. adrenal glands
   d. pancreas

5. What lymph nodes are located surrounding the major blood vessels of the retroperitoneum?
   a. visceral lymph nodes
   b. parietal lymph nodes
   c. superficial abdominal nodes
   d. axillary lymph nodes

6. Parietal nodes can be found in the retroperitoneum do NOT surround which of the following vessel?
   a. portal vein
   b. celiac axis
   c. internal iliac artery
   d. superior mesenteric artery

7. What lymph nodes are located along the small bowel and mesentery?
   a. Chyle cistern nodes
   b. parietal nodes
   c. visceral nodes
   d. lacteals

8. Lymph nodes affected by lymphadenitis typically do NOT have which of the following characteristics?
   a. ovoid shape
   b. loss of the fatty hilum
   c. hyperemia
   d. larger than normal

9. Primary malignant lymph nodes do NOT have which of the following characteristics?
   a. more hypoechoic
   b. round shape
   c. loss of the fatty hilum
   d. hyperemia

10. Which of the following statements regarding lymphadenopathy and AIDS is FALSE?
    a. Enlarged lymph nodes appear hyperechoic with a loss of the fatty hilum.
    b. Enlarged lymph nodes appear hypoechoic and bowel wall thickening may also be seen.
    c. Lymph nodes in patients with tuberculosis may appear anechoic due to necrosis.
    d. Patients with AIDS may develop Kaposi sarcoma and lymphoma.

11. Which of the following is NOT a malignant tumor of the retroperitoneum?
    a. liposarcoma
    b. rhabdomyosarcoma
    c. myxosarcoma
    d. retroperitoneal fibrosis

12. What is the most common primary malignancy of the retroperitoneum?
    a. liposarcoma
    b. rhabdomyosarcoma
    c. myxosarcoma
    d. retroperitoneal fibrosis

13. What is the sonographic appearance of liposarcomas?
    a. extremely large, poorly marginated, complex retroperitoneal mass
    b. large, well-defined hyperechoic mass
    c. small, well-defined hyperechoic mass
    d. large echogenic mass that tends to infiltrate surrounding structures such as the IVC

14. What is the most common site for retroperitoneal infections?
    a. anterior pararenal space
    b. posterior pararenal space
    c. perirenal space
    d. perinephric space

15. What is the most common cause of posterior pararenal fluid collections?
    a. urinoma from urinary system rupture
    b. abscess or hemorrhage from aortic disease
    c. abscess from appendicitis or Crohn's disease
    d. lymphocele from renal transplant

16. Your patient presents with a history of pancreatitis to rule out the presence of a pseudocyst. Which retroperitoneal compartment would contain a pseudocyst?
    a. anterior pararenal space
    b. posterior pararenal space
    c. perirenal space
    d. perinephric space

17. A patient presents with a history of left ureteropelvic junction obstruction. A fluid collection is seen surrounding the left kidney. What is the likely diagnosis of the fluid collection?
    a. hematoma
    b. urinoma
    c. lymphocele
    d. abscess

18. While performing an abdominal examination on a patient, you suspect the lymph nodes surrounding the great vessels are enlarged. What is the normal measurement for the lymph nodes in this location?
    a. less than 5 mm
    b. less than 7 mm
    c. less than 10 mm
    d. less than 20 mm

19. Which retroperitoneal compartment contains the psoas and quadratus lumborum muscles?
    a. anterior pararenal space
    b. posterior pararenal space
    c. perirenal space
    d. perinephric space

20. While performing an abdominal sonogram you notice multiple rounded hypoechoic structures in the splenic and left renal hilum. These structures appear to be distorting the surrounding blood vessels. What is the most likely diagnosis?
    a. abscess
    b. lymphocele
    c. lymphadenopathy
    d. retroperitoneal fibrosis

Fill-in-the-Blank

1. The area that lies behind the _____ is referred to as the retroperitoneum. The retroperitoneum lies between the _____ and anterior to the _____.

2. The retroperitoneum is divided into three major compartments by the _____ and _____ _____ fascia. The anterior renal fascia is also referred to as _____ fascia and the posterior renal fascia is referred to as _____ fascia.

3. The anterior pararenal space is bordered anteriorly by the posterior _____ _____ and posteriorly by the anterior _____ _____.

4. The perirenal space is bordered anteriorly by the _____ _____ _____ and posteriorly by the _____ _____ _____.

5. The posterior pararenal space lies between the _____ _____ fascia and the _____ fascia. The _____ muscles and the _____ _____ muscles are located within this space.

6. The _____ _____ is a dilated collecting area that is located in the mid-retroperitoneum and collects lymph from the lower extremities and pelvis before ascending to the _____ duct.

7. Lymph nodes are located 360 degrees around the great vessels. The nodes that lie posterior to the great vessels may displace the aorta and IVC _____ when enlarged.

8. _____ is the term for enlargement of the lymph nodes due to _____, _____, or _____.

9. An enlargement of lymph nodes due to an inflammatory process is called _____.

10. Retroperitoneal fibrosis, also called _____ disease, can encase the _____, _____, and _____ of the retroperitoneum. If the ureters are affected, _____ can occur.

11. Malignant tumors tend to be _____ and more _____ than their benign counterparts. Retroperitoneal tumors demonstrate a _____ on surrounding structures.

12. The second most common primary retroperitoneal malignancy is _____. Differential diagnoses include _____, _____, and _____ malignancy.

13. Retroperitoneal fluid collections include _____, _____, _____, and _____.

14. Fluid collections within the perirenal space are generally associated with _____ abnormalities. Sonographically, fluid is contained within the borders of the renal _____.

15. A _____ is a fluid collection that may occur following lymph node dissection for cancer staging.

Short Answer

1. List the major functions of the lymphatic system. What role do the lymph nodes play?

2. The psoas and quadratus lumborum muscles can be mistaken for a fluid collection in certain patients. What techniques can be used to ensure that these structures are normal?

3. If a mass or fluid collection is identified within the retroperitoneum, what should the sonographer document in a complete examination?

4. Sonographically, how can one distinguish between lymph nodes enlarged from inflammation and those enlarged due to malignancy?

5. Why do retroperitoneal masses typically go undiagnosed for so long?

IMAGE EVALUATION/PATHOLOGY

Review the images and answer the following questions.

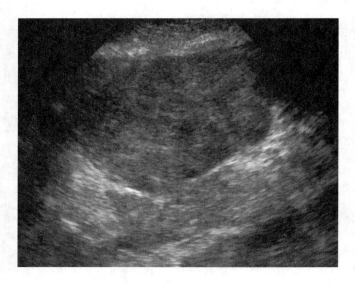

1. A 44-year-old patient presents with abdominal pain and distention. Describe the mass seen in the retroperitoneal cavity of this patient. List the possible differential diagnoses for a solid retroperitoneal mass that appears separate from the kidneys and adrenal glands.

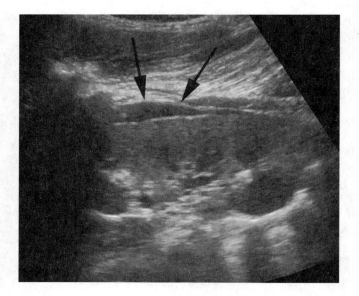

2. This patient had a left renal biopsy done earlier today and complains of worsening left flank pain. Describe what is seen in this image. What is the likely diagnosis?

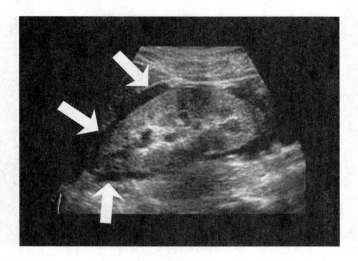

3. A 52-year-old patient presents with a history of bladder outlet obstruction, fever, and hydronephrosis. The patient complains of bilateral flank pain and nausea. This image was taken in the left upper quadrant. What are the *arrows* pointing to? What is the most likely diagnosis?

CASE STUDY

Review the image and answer the following questions.

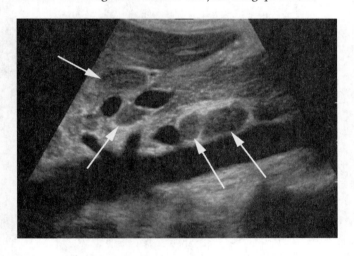

1. This image was taken in a 45-year-old man who has a long-standing history of AIDS. What are the *arrows* in this image pointing to? Do the structures appear normal? Where are the structures located? What is the likely diagnosis?

PART TWO

SUPERFICIAL STRUCTURE SONOGRAPHY

The Thyroid Gland, Parathyroid Glands, and Neck

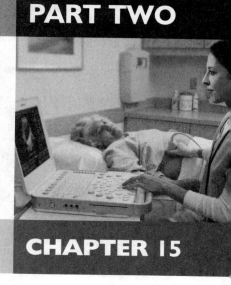

CHAPTER 15

REVIEW OF GLOSSARY TERMS

Matching

Match the terms with their definitions.

KEY TERMS

1. _____ adenoma

2. _____ adenopathy

3. _____ anaplasia

4. _____ cold nodule

5. _____ euthyroid

6. _____ fine-needle aspiration

7. _____ goiter

8. _____ Graves disease

9. _____ Hashimoto thyroiditis

10. _____ heterotopic

11. _____ hyperparathyroidism

12. _____ hypophosphatasia

13. _____ hypothyroidism

14. _____ indolent

15. _____ isthmus

16. _____ longus colli muscles

17. _____ microcalcifications

DEFINITION

a. Focal or diffuse thyroid gland enlargement due to iodine deficiency

b. Most common form of thyroid cancer

c. Inflammation of the thyroid

d. Underactive thyroid hormones

e. Thyroid gland is producing the right amount of thyroid hormone

f. Increase in color Doppler vascular flow in the thyroid

g. Enlargement of the glands

h. Wedge-shaped muscle posterior to the thyroid lobes

i. Occurring at an abnormal place or upon the wrong part of the body

j. Sternohyoid and sternothyroid muscles located anterior to the thyroid

k. Invasive procedure using a small gauge needle to obtain a tissue specimen from a specific lesion

l. Hyperechoic foci that may or may not shadow

m. Low phosphatase level that can be seen with hyperparathyroidism

n. Benign solid tumor

o. Loss of differentiation of cells, which is characteristic of tumor tissue

p. Hormone produced by the parathyroid glands that regulates serum calcium and phosphorus

q. Congenital anomaly located anterior to trachea, extending from the base of the tongue to the isthmus of the thyroid

r. Hormone secreted by the anterior pituitary gland that stimulates the thyroid gland to secrete T4 and T3

s. Large muscles located anterolateral to the thyroid

t. Area seen on nuclear medicine study as a region of thyroid where the radioisotope has not been taken up

(*Continued on page 140*)

KEY TERMS

18. _____ papillary carcinoma

19. _____ parathyroid hormone

20. _____ primary hyperparathyroidism

21. _____ sternocleidomastoid muscles

22. _____ strap muscles

23. _____ thyroiditis

24. _____ thyroglossal duct cyst

25. _____ thyroid inferno

26. _____ thyroid-stimulating hormone

DEFINITION

u. An autoimmune hyperthyroidism caused by antibodies that continuously activate TSH receptors

v. Oversecretion of parathyroid hormones

w. Disorder associated with elevated serum calcium levels, usually caused by benign parathyroid adenoma

x. Causing little pain or slow growing

y. The band of thyroid tissue connecting the right and left lobes

z. Most common inflammatory disease of the thyroid gland

ANATOMY AND PHYSIOLOGY REVIEW

Image Labeling

Complete the labels in the images that follow.

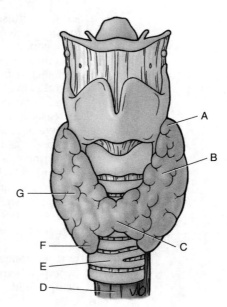

1. Anterior view of the neck

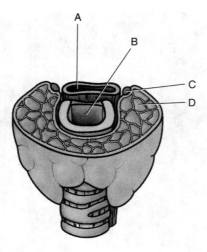

2. Anterosuperior view of the neck

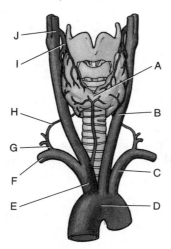

3. Arterial vasculature of the neck

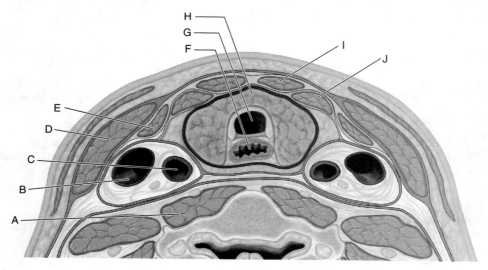

4. Musculature of the neck

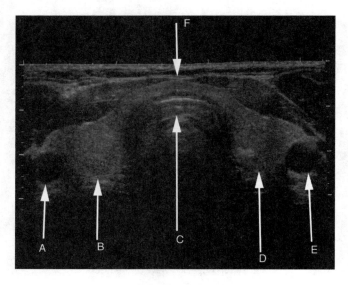

5. Sonographic anatomy

CHAPTER REVIEW

Multiple Choice

Complete each question by circling the best answer.

1. Which of the following transducers would be appropriate for evaluation of the thyroid gland and neck on an average patient?

   a. 7.5 MHz curvilinear
   b. 5 MHz phased array
   c. 5 MHz linear array
   d. 12 MHz linear array

2. The thyroid and parathyroid both have what common function?

   a. endocrine glands
   b. exocrine glands
   c. sebaceous glands
   d. apocrine glands

3. What is the main function of the thyroid gland?

   a. production of calcium
   b. storage of fats and vitamins
   c. regulation of the basal metabolic rate
   d. production of antibodies

4. Which of the following regarding the anatomy of the neck and thyroid gland is FALSE?

   a. The strap muscles are anterolateral to the thyroid gland.
   b. The longus colli muscle is seen posterior to the thyroid gland.
   c. The trachea forms the lateral border of the thyroid gland.
   d. The common carotid artery and internal jugular vein are posterolateral to the thyroid gland.

5. Which of the following is NOT a strap muscle?

   a. sternothyroid muscle
   b. sternohyoid muscle
   c. sternocleidomastoid muscle
   d. omohyoid muscle

6. A radioiodine scintigraphy examination can be used to evaluate thyroid nodules. Which of the following statements regarding this examination is FALSE?

   a. Nodules may be classified as either hot or cold nodules.
   b. A hot nodule traps an excessive amount of isotope and is hyperfunctioning.
   c. A cold nodule does not absorb the isotope and demonstrates an area of decreased or absent activity.
   d. All cold nodules are malignant.

7. Which of the following is NOT a typical symptom of Graves disease?

   a. hyperthyroidism
   b. elevated levels of T3 and T4
   c. a shrunken echogenic thyroid gland
   d. bulging of the eyes

8. What is the most common functional disorder of the thyroid gland?

   a. hyperthyroidism
   b. thyrotoxicosis
   c. Graves disease
   d. hypothyroidism

9. A patient presents for evaluation of the thyroid gland with a history of Hashimoto thyroiditis. Which of the following is NOT a common symptom of this condition?
   a. weight loss
   b. cold intolerance
   c. menstrual irregularities
   d. fatigue

10. On sonographic examination, your patient presents with an enlarged heterogeneous thyroid gland. The patient's lab work is normal, and the patient is not experiencing any symptoms besides the palpable, enlarged gland. What is the most likely diagnosis?
    a. multinodular goiter
    b. Graves disease
    c. Hashimoto thyroiditis
    d. thyrotoxicosis

11. What is the most common form of thyroid cancer?
    a. follicular
    b. papillary
    c. medullary
    d. anaplastic

12. Which of the following characteristics increases the suspicion for malignancy in a thyroid nodule?
    a. eggshell calcifications
    b. hyperechogenicity
    c. microcalcifications
    d. peripheral calcifications

13. Which of the following is NOT a characteristic of benign thyroid nodules?
    a. a uniform hypoechoic halo
    b. avascularity
    c. well-defined, regular margins
    d. taller-than-wide shape

14. Which of the following is NOT a characteristic of a metastatic lymph node?
    a. increasing size on serial examinations
    b. microcalcifications
    c. prominent fatty hilum
    d. rounded, bulging shape

15. Which type of thyroid cancer is seen in patients with a personal history of multiple endocrine neoplasia type 2 syndrome?
    a. papillary carcinoma
    b. medullary carcinoma
    c. follicular carcinoma
    d. anaplastic carcinoma

16. Which aggressive form of thyroid cancer has a tendency to compress and destroy the local structures of the neck?
    a. papillary carcinoma
    b. medullary carcinoma
    c. follicular carcinoma
    d. anaplastic carcinoma

17. Fine-needle aspiration is NOT effective for diagnosing which form of thyroid carcinoma?
    a. papillary carcinoma
    b. medullary carcinoma
    c. follicular carcinoma
    d. anaplastic carcinoma

18. How many parathyroid glands do most adults have?
    a. 2
    b. 4
    c. 6
    d. 8

19. What is the most common cause of primary hyperparathyroidism?
    a. breast or prostate cancer
    b. chronic renal insufficiency
    c. parathyroid carcinoma
    d. parathyroid adenoma

20. While performing an examination of the thyroid gland, a small, solid, oval, homogeneously hypoechoic mass is seen posterior to the mid-lateral lobe of the thyroid gland. This appears to be separate from the thyroid gland. What is the most likely diagnosis?
    a. hyperplasia of the parathyroid glands
    b. parathyroid adenoma
    c. papillary carcinoma
    d. multinodular goiter

Fill-in-the-Blank

1. The thyroid is an _____ gland that is made up of a _____ and _____ lobe, connected by a thin _____ of tissue.

2. The mean length of the thyroid gland is _____, mean AP diameter is _____, and mean thickness of the isthmus is _____.

3. The thyroid gland receives a rich blood supply from four arteries: the paired _____ _____ _____, which arise from the external carotids, and the _____ _____ _____, which originate at the thyrocervical trunk of the subclavian artery.

4. The _____ and _____ thyroid veins drain into the IJV, whereas the _____ thyroid veins drain into the brachiocephalic veins.

5. The common carotid artery and internal jugular vein form the _____ _____ border of the thyroid gland. The _____ _____ muscle is seen posterior to the gland.

6. The thyroid gland secretes three hormones: _____, _____, and _____. _____ is needed to properly synthesize the hormones.

7. Maintenance of the concentrations of T3 and T4 is controlled by a regulatory system that involves the _____, the _____, and the thyroid gland.

8. A condition that is associated with excessive release of thyroid hormones is called _____, whereas one associated with a thyroid hormone deficiency is referred to as _____.

9. The echotexture of the normal thyroid gland is _____, and _____ when compared to the adjacent musculature.

10. Congenital cysts of the neck include _____ _____ _____, which tend to be midline, and _____ _____ _____, which tend to lie lateral to the carotid artery.

11. Thyroid adenomas are benign nodules contained within a _____ _____. A minority of adenomas are toxic and cause _____. Typically, an adenoma will demonstrate a _____ _____ surrounding the nodule. Sonographically, large adenomas have the characteristics of a _____ _____.

12. A nontoxic goiter refers to an enlargement of the entire gland without evidence of discrete _____ and without _____ disturbance. Simple goiters may convert into _____ goiters, demonstrated by a multilobulated, asymmetrically enlarged gland.

13. _____ is a hypermetabolic state caused by elevated levels of free _____ and _____. The majority of patients with hyperthyroidism have _____ disease, which is an _____ disease.

14. The most common cause of primary hypothyroidism is _____ _____.

15. Malignant thyroid nodules are typically solid and _____ when compared to the normal thyroid parenchyma. The presence of _____ is one of the most specific sonographic features of thyroid malignancy. They are commonly found in _____ thyroid cancer.

16. Papillary carcinoma most commonly occurs between the ages of _____, and it is three times more common in _____.

17. A definitive diagnosis of papillary carcinoma can be made by _____ _____ _____.
    The overall survival rate of this type of thyroid cancer is _____, making it the least aggressive form of
    thyroid cancer.

18. Most adults have _____ parathyroid glands: two _____ located posterior to the mid-portion
    of the thyroid gland and two _____ located in a more variable position.

19. The parathyroid glands are responsible for producing _____ _____, which regulates the con-
    centrations of _____ and _____.

20. Primary hyperplasia is enlargement of _____ _____ _____ and should be ex-
    pected when _____ nodules are identified, whereas _____ _____ should be sus-
    pected when a solitary nodule is identified.

Short Answer

1. Give three causes of primary hyperthyroidism. List five clinical symptoms of hyperthyroidism.

2. What is the most common cause of primary hypothyroidism? List five clinical symptoms of hypothyroidism.

3. Describe the technique used to perform a fine-needle aspiration of a suspicious thyroid nodule.

4. You are asked to evaluate the parathyroid glands during a sonographic examination of the neck. What landmarks
   will you use to locate the parathyroid glands?

5. What is the most common cause of hyperparathyroidism? List five clinical symptoms of hyperparathyroidism.

IMAGE EVALUATION/PATHOLOGY

Review the images and answer the following questions.

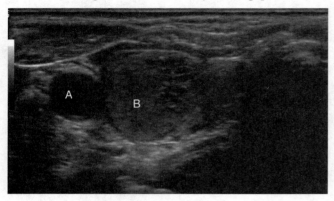

1. Identify the structure labeled "*A.*" Describe the mass labeled "*B.*"

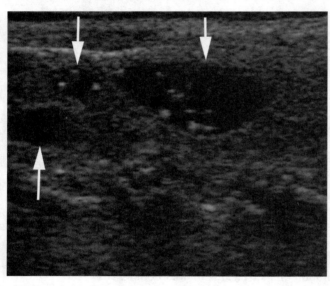

2. Describe the three nodules indicated by *arrows* in this sagittal image of the thyroid gland. What two characteristics in these lesions are suspicious for malignancy?

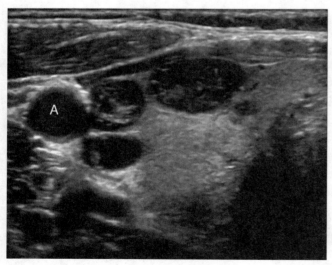

3. Describe the three lesions seen in this transverse image of the thyroid gland. List two characteristics in these lesions that are associated with a low risk for malignancy.

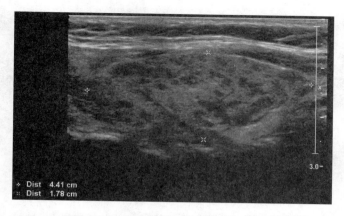

4. This patient presents with an enlarged thyroid on physical examination. Her laboratory values revealed hypothyroidism. Describe the thyroid gland seen in this image. What is the most common cause of hypothyroidism and the most likely diagnosis?

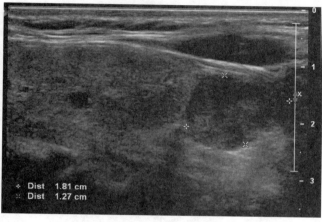

5. Describe the mass measured in this image. This mass is inferior to the thyroid gland and appears to be separate from the thyroid tissue. What is the most likely diagnosis? What symptoms might this cause?

CASE STUDIES

Review the images and answer the following questions.

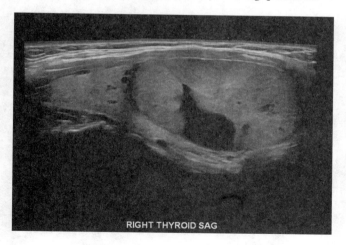

RIGHT THYROID SAG

1. This patient presents with a large palpable mass in the right neck. The patient's laboratory workup was normal. Describe the thyroid seen in this sagittal image. How would a definitive diagnosis for this lesion be made?

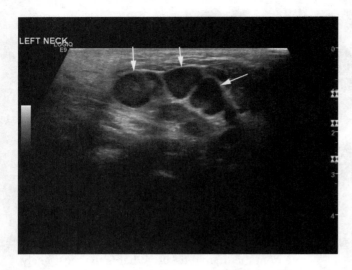

2. This patient presents with a tender palpable neck mass. This image was taken lateral and superior to the left thyroid gland. What structures are the *arrows* pointing to? What can cause this appearance?

The Breast

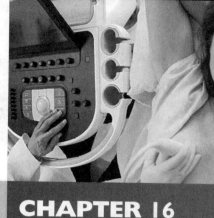

REVIEW OF GLOSSARY TERMS

Matching

Match the terms with their definitions.

KEY TERMS

1. _____ adenopathy

2. _____ areola

3. _____ axilla

4. _____ BIRADS

5. _____ Cooper's ligaments

6. _____ desmoplastic reaction

7. _____ echopalpation

8. _____ elastography

9. _____ in situ

10. _____ multicentric breast cancer

11. _____ multifocal breast cancer

12. _____ sentinel node

13. _____ spiculation

14. _____ TDLU

DEFINITION

a. Fingerlike extension of a malignant tumor

b. Technique used to locate a palpable mass with sonography

c. Pigmented skin surrounding the nipple

d. Coexistent cancers within different quadrants or separated by more than 5 cm within the breast

e. First node in the drainage basin and at most risk for metastasis

f. Enlarged lymph nodes

g. Technique that compares the relative stiffness of a mass compared to the adjacent tissues

h. Armpit, significant because it contains the lymph nodes that drain the breast tissue

i. Functional unit of the breast, composed of a lobule and its draining extralobular terminal duct

j. Thin connective tissue bands that connect breast tissue to the skin and provide structural support to the breast

k. Breast imaging and reporting data system published by the ACR in an effort to promote the use of more consistent terminology

l. Noninvasive breast cancer

m. The presence of additional malignant lesions within a breast quadrant or within 5 cm of the primary tumor, indicating the spread of cancer via the ducts

n. Fibroelastic, reactive fibrosis that occurs in the tissues surrounding many malignant breast lesions

ANATOMY AND PHYSIOLOGY REVIEW

Image Labeling

Complete the labels in the images that follow.

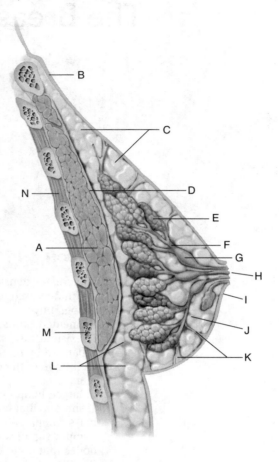

1. Breast anatomy

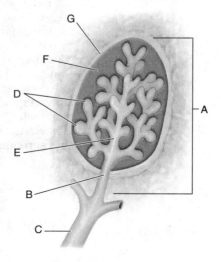

2. Functional unit of the breast

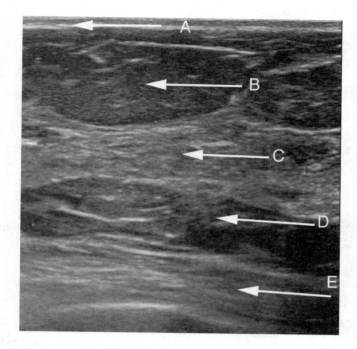

3. Zonal anatomy of the breast

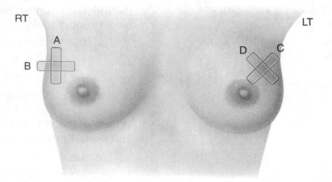

TRANSDUCER SCAN PLANES

4. Transducer scan planes

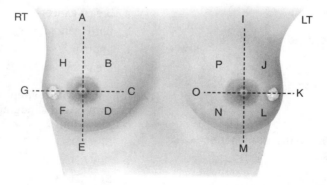

QUADRANT AND CLOCK-FACE ANNOTATION

5. Quadrant and clock-face annotation

CHAPTER REVIEW

Multiple Choice

Complete each question by circling the best answer.

1. Which of the following statements regarding mammography is FALSE?
   a. Mammography cannot determine whether a mass is cystic or solid.
   b. Mammography can be difficult in patients who have inflammatory conditions or trauma to the breast.
   c. Mammography can easily detect lesions in a dense breast.
   d. Mammography can detect microcalcifications, which may be the first sign of a malignancy.

2. Which of the following statements regarding breast sonography is FALSE?
   a. Sonography is useful for differentiating cystic from solid lesions.
   b. Sonography is often used to guide interventional and therapeutic procedures.
   c. Sonography can be used to evaluate the male breast.
   d. Sonography is as good as mammography in detecting microcalcifications.

3. What is the functional unit of the breast?
   a. radial ductal unit
   b. terminal ductal lobular unit
   c. stromal ductal unit
   d. glandular ductal unit

4. Where is the majority of the glandular tissue of the breast found?
   a. upper outer quadrant
   b. upper inner quadrant
   c. lower outer quadrant
   d. lower inner quadrant

5. What attaches the breast tissue to the skin?
   a. TDLUs
   b. lactiferous ligaments
   c. Cooper's ligaments
   d. thoracic ligaments

6. The majority of breast lymph drains into what nodes?
   a. internal mammary nodes
   b. axillary nodes
   c. rotter nodes
   d. thoracic nodes

7. Which breast layer is located between the anterior and posterior mammary fascia?
   a. subcutaneous fat layer
   b. mammary layer
   c. retromammary fat layer
   d. axilla

8. An intramammary lymph node is identified during a breast sonography examination. What is the normal measurement of an intramammary lymph node?
   a. less than 5 mm
   b. less than 1 cm
   c. less than 2 cm
   d. normal lymph nodes are not visualized within the breast

9. According to ACR and AIUM guidelines, which of the following transducers is appropriate to use for breast sonography?
   a. 7.5 MHz linear array
   b. 7.5 MHz phased array
   c. 12 MHz linear array
   d. 15 MHz curvilinear array

10. Which of the following can help improve contrast and spatial resolution during breast sonography?
    a. harmonic imaging
    b. spatial compounding
    c. broad bandwidth transducers
    d. all the above are used to improve image quality

11. What is the most common cause of breast lumps in women 35 to 50 years of age?
    a. breast cancers
    b. fibroadenomas
    c. lipomas
    d. breast cysts

12. A patient with a simple cyst seen on both mammography and sonography would be given which classification?
    a. BI-RADS 1
    b. BI-RADS 2
    c. BI-RADS 3
    d. BI-RADS 4

13. A patient presents for breast sonography after a lesion was seen on a mammogram. A cyst that does not meet all the criteria for a simple cyst is found that correlates to the area seen on mammography. Which of the following characteristics would NOT be worrisome for malignancy or neoplastic changes?

    a. thickened cyst wall > 5 mm

    b. a mixed cystic or solid lesion

    c. a fluid-debris level that changes with patient positioning

    d. echoes along the wall of the cyst that do not change with patient positioning

14. What is the name of a retention cyst that may develop in pregnant or lactating women?

    a. papillary apocrine metaplasia

    b. sebaceous cyst

    c. epidermal inclusion cyst

    d. galactocele

15. A patient presents with a history of breast surgery to remove a benign lesion. While scanning over the incision site, you suspect you are imaging the postsurgical scar. What is the typical sonographic appearance of a scar?

    a. hypoechoic area with acoustic shadowing that is reduced or eliminated with transducer pressure

    b. hyperechoic area with acoustic shadowing that is reduced or eliminated with transducer pressure

    c. hypoechoic area with acoustic shadowing that remains constant regardless of transducer pressure or angulation

    d. hypoechoic area with hyperemia seen with color Doppler

16. What is the most common benign solid tumor of the female breast?

    a. phyllodes tumor

    b. intraductal papilloma

    c. lipoma

    d. fibroadenoma

17. What is the most common noninvasive breast cancer?

    a. LCIS

    b. DCIS

    c. IDC NOS

    d. ILC

18. Which of the following is an uncommon cancer that presents with redness and eczema-like crusting of the nipple and areola, nipple discharge, and itching?

    a. Mondor disease

    b. Ormond disease

    c. Paget disease

    d. medullary disease

19. What is the most common breast cancer?

    a. LCIS

    b. DCIS

    c. IDC NOS

    d. ILC

20. What is the most common male breast abnormality?

    a. fibroadenoma

    b. simple cyst

    c. breast cancer

    d. gynecomastia

21. Which of the following statements regarding elastography of the breast is TRUE?

    a. Hard lesions tend to show more deformation or strain than soft tissues.

    b. A cancer will tend to be larger on the elastogram than on the conventional 2D image.

    c. Most benign masses tend to be stiffer on elastography.

    d. A cancer will tend to be smaller on the elastogram than on the conventional 2D image.

22. Which of the following is NOT a sonographic characteristic of a benign mass?

    a. A benign mass displaces rather than invades surrounding tissues.

    b. A benign mass is typically well circumscribed.

    c. A benign mass is typically taller than wide.

    d. A benign mass typically has an oval shape.

23. Which of the following characteristics make a mass suspicious for malignancy?

    a. angular or spiculated margins

    b. nipple retraction

    c. shadowing

    d. all of the above are suspicious findings

24. A mass that is highly suggestive of malignancy on both mammography and sonography with multiple suspicious features would be classified as what?

    a. BI-RADS 2

    b. BI-RADS 3

    c. BI-RADS 4

    d. BI-RADS 5

25. Which type of breast cancer begins in the ducts and does not invade the basement membrane?

    a. LCIS

    b. DCIS

    c. IDC NOS

    d. ILC

Fill-in-the-Blank

1. _____ is the most commonly used imaging modality to evaluate the breast and remains the only widely used screening tool proven to reduce breast cancer mortality.

2. Mammography is capable of detecting suspicious patterns of _____, which is typically the first imaging sign of a developing malignancy. Lesions are more readily detected in a radiolucent or _____ breast than in a radiopaque or _____ breast.

3. Sonography can help differentiate _____ from _____ lesions. Sonography can also be useful in patients who are _____, _____, or _____, because these patients tend to have increased breast density that can limit the radiographic examination.

4. The breast is subdivided by fascial planes into three layers: the _____ _____ layer, the _____ layer, and the _____ _____ layer.

5. Within the mammary layer are _____ overlapping lobes arranged in a _____ fashion around the nipple. Each lobe contains _____ TDLUs.

6. The _____ major muscle lies beneath the upper two-thirds of the breast. The _____ _____ muscle lies beneath the major muscle.

7. Normal skin thickness in the breast is _____ or less, but it can be slightly thicker near the _____ and _____ _____.

8. The _____ _____ layer lies between the posterior mammary fascia and the pectoralis major muscle.

9. When evaluating the breast, sagittal and transverse planes can be used as well as _____ and _____ planes.

10. Image annotations should include the side being examined, _____ in the breast, and transducer _____ _____. Distance from the _____ is also recommended by the ACR.

11. In mammography, the CC or _____ view demonstrates the _____, central, and _____ breast. The MLO or _____ _____ _____ view demonstrates the breast in profile from the _____ to the _____ fold and includes a portion of the _____ muscle.

12. The most common benign diffuse breast condition is _____ _____. Symptoms include breast _____, fullness, and _____. With sonography, multiple breast _____ are commonly seen.

13. Inflammation of the breast is called _____ and it most commonly occurs in women who are _____ or _____. Without treatment, an _____ may develop.

14. A condition that is the result of inflammatory and ischemic processes, frequently the consequence of breast trauma, is called _____ _____. Sonographically, initially there may be _____

echogenicity at the palpable area. An _____ _____ may form as a result displaying a fat-fluid level.

15. A palpable, oval, well-circumscribed, solid mass that is enlarging in pregnancy is commonly a secretory or _____ _____.

16. An intraductal papilloma typically occurs within a major _____ _____. This lesion may cause _____ of the duct, leading to cyst formation.

17. Approximately one in _____ women will develop breast cancer in their lifetime. The majority occur in women over the age of _____. Most cancers originate in a _____. Because it has the highest percentage of glandular and epithelial tissue, the _____ _____ quadrant is the most likely location for a breast cancer to develop.

18. Noninvasive breast cancer is called carcinoma _____. Types include _____ _____ _____ and _____ _____ _____.

19. Invasive cancer describes cases when malignant cells breach the _____ _____ of the duct and/or lobule and extend into adjacent tissues. _____ _____ _____ _____ is the most common breast cancer.

20. When IDC NOS is palpable, it typically is _____, _____, and _____. Lesions with _____ _____ can feel larger on palpation than their actual size due to the response of the surrounding tissues.

21. Invasive lobular carcinoma is more often _____, _____, and bilateral than invasive ductal carcinoma. _____ is not a typical feature with ILC, as it is with IDC.

22. A clinical symptom of papillary carcinoma is _____ _____ _____.

23. _____ carcinoma occurs when a highly invasive cancer infiltrates the lymphatics of the skin. The skin becomes _____, _____, and _____ with an orange peel appearance.

24. The first site of metastatic spread from a primary breast cancer is usually to the _____ _____ lymph nodes. The _____ node is the first node in the drainage basin at most risk for metastasis. Distant sites for metastasis include _____, _____, _____, and _____.

25. Vocal _____ is a technique using power Doppler in which a patient is asked to hum during real-time imaging. Abnormal tissues will tend to show a _____ of color during this technique.

Short Answer

1. Mammography remains the most widely used screening tool in breast imaging. Discuss the advantages and drawbacks of mammography.

2. Sonography plays an important role in evaluating the breast as well. List four indications for breast sonography and four advantages of breast sonography.

3. Describe the common patient positioning techniques used during breast sonography. How are the images typically labeled?

4. Describe the sonographic characteristics that make a mass suspicious for malignancy.

5. Breast sonography can be used to evaluate breast implants. List three common complications that occur with breast implant surgery and describe their sonographic appearance.

IMAGE EVALUATION/PATHOLOGY

Review the images and answer the following questions.

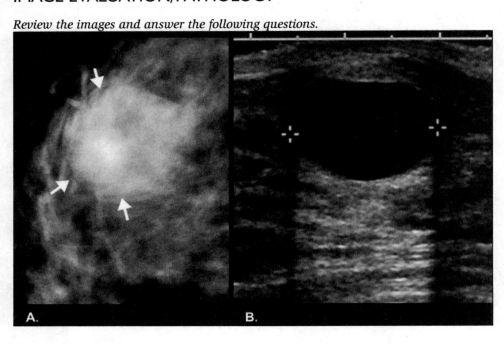

1. List the sonographic characteristics of a simple breast cyst, seen here in this image.

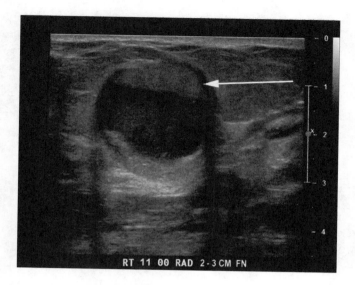

RT 11 00 RAD 2-3 CM FN

2. This image of a galactocele was seen in a 32-year-old woman who was breast-feeding. Describe the mass. What is the *arrow* pointing to? According to the annotation on the image, what quadrant of the breast is this mass located in?

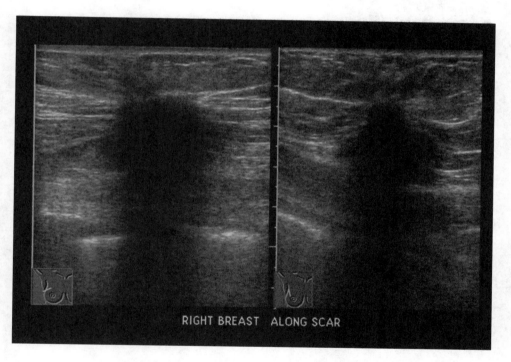

RIGHT BREAST ALONG SCAR

3. This image was taken over a surgical scar. What characteristics are seen that are suspicious for malignancy? What characteristic is seen that is indicative of a surgical scar? What techniques can help distinguish a scar from a recurrent tumor?

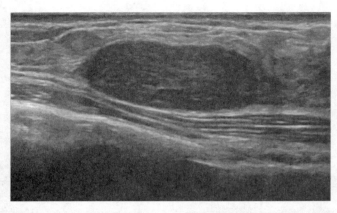

4. This palpable mass was found in a 32-year-old female. Describe the characteristics of the mass. What is the likely diagnosis?

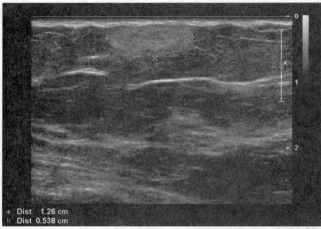

5. Describe the mass marked by the calipers. If this palpable mass is located in the left breast at 11:00, which quadrant is it located in?

CASE STUDIES

Review the images and answer the following questions.

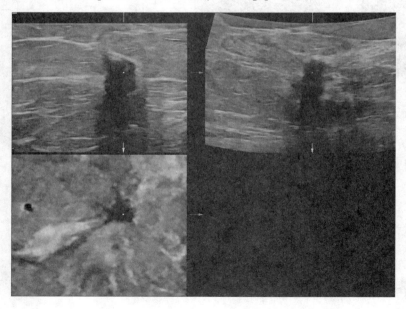

1. A 49-year-old woman presented for her routine mammogram and a suspicious area was noted in the left breast. A follow-up sonography examination was ordered, and this lesion was noted at 1:00. What technique was used to create this image? What suspicious characteristics are noted? What quadrant is the mass located in?

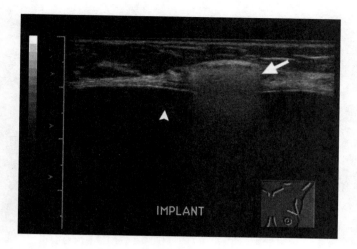

2. A 44-year-old patient with a history of breast augmentation with silicone implants presents with a palpable lump in the left outer quadrant. What does the large arrow represent? What is this sign called? Is this an intracapsular or extracapsular rupture?

The Scrotum

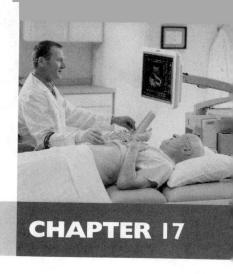

REVIEW OF GLOSSARY TERMS

Matching

Match the terms with their definitions.

KEY TERMS

1. _____ AFP

2. _____ beta-hCG

3. _____ cryptorchidism

4. _____ hyperemia

5. _____ infarction

6. _____ orchiopexy

7. _____ pampiniform plexus

8. _____ Valsalva maneuver

DEFINITION

a. Surgical procedure done to fasten an undescended testicle into the scrotum or repair an acute testicular torsion

b. Undescended testicle

c. Alpha fetoprotein level that may be elevated with hepatocellular carcinoma and certain testicular cancers

d. A technique in which the patient is asked to bear down to increase the intra-abdominal pressure and aid in the diagnosis of varicocele and scrotal hernia

e. An increase in blood flow to the tissue

f. Tissue death that occurs due to a lack of blood flow

g. A network of veins that drains the epididymis and testis

h. Human chorionic gonadotropin is produced during pregnancy but is also secreted by certain testicular cancers

ANATOMY AND PHYSIOLOGY REVIEW

Image Labeling

Complete the labels in the images that follow.

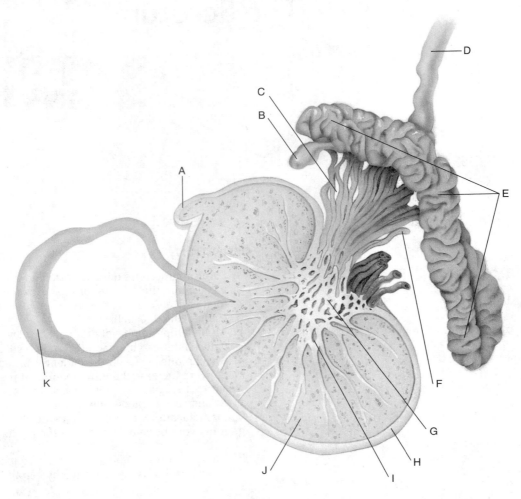

1. Scrotal anatomy

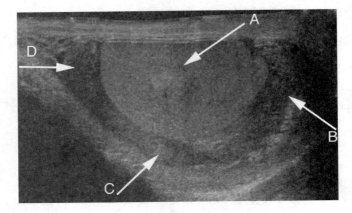

2. Scrotal anatomy

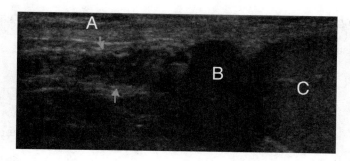

3. Scrotal anatomy

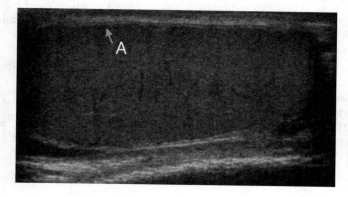

4. Scrotal anatomy

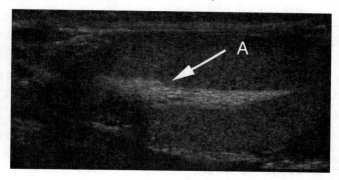

5. Scrotal anatomy

CHAPTER REVIEW

Multiple Choice

Complete each question by circling the best answer.

1. You receive a request to evaluate a child with a history of undescended testis. Where are the majority of undescended testes located?

   a. in the contralateral scrotum

   b. in the flank area near the kidney

   c. in the abdominal cavity

   d. in the inguinal canal

2. Which of the following is NOT located within the scrotum?

   a. testes

   b. seminal vesicles

   c. spermatic cord

   d. epididymis

3. While performing a sonographic examination of the scrotum, you suspect a varicocele is present. What is the normal measurement of the veins in the pampiniform plexus?

   a. less than 1 mm

   b. less than 2 mm

   c. less than 5 mm

   d. less than 1 cm

4. Which of the following is NOT part of the anatomical division of the epididymis?

   a. tail

   b. body

   c. neck

   d. head

5. While obtaining a patient's history, you learn that he has had a vasectomy. Which of the following scrotal pathologies is NOT more common in patients who have had a vasectomy?

   a. spermatocele

   b. epididymal cyst

   c. seminoma

   d. dilatation of the rete testis

6. Which of the following is the fibrous sheath that covers and protects the testis and also makes up the mediastinum testis?

   a. tunica albuginea

   b. tunica vaginalis

   c. tunica gubernaculum

   d. tunica parietalis

7. Which of the following undergoes tubular ectasia caused by dilatation of the seminiferous tubules and is associated with epididymal cysts and spermatoceles?

   a. mediastinum testis

   b. rete testis

   c. tunica vaginalis

   d. tunica albuginea

   e. dilatation of the seminiferous tubules is refered to as *tubular ectasia* of the rete testis. This is often seen bilaterally and is associated with epididymal cysts and spermatoceles

8. Which of the following statements regarding the testicular veins is FALSE?

   a. The testis is drained by the veins of the pampiniform plexus.

   b. The veins of the pampiniform plexus empty into the testicular veins.

   c. The right testicular vein drains directly into the IVC.

   d. The left testicular vein drains directly into the IVC.

9. A patient with a history of undescended testis is NOT at an increased risk for which of the following?

   a. seminoma

   b. testicular torsion

   c. infertility

   d. teratoma

10. What is the most common cause of acute scrotal pain?

    a. testicular torsion

    b. testicular malignancy

    c. epididymitis and epididymo-orchitis

    d. scrotal hernia

11. Between what ages is testicular torsion most common?

    a. 6 to 12 years of age

    b. 12 to 18 years of age

    c. 22 to 30 years of age

    d. 40 to 50 years of age

12. In young men, what is most common cause of epididymitis?

    a. sexually transmitted disease

    b. scrotal trauma

    c. torsion

    d. infertility

13. What is a collection of serous fluid located between the layers of the tunica vaginalis called?

    a. tunica albuginea cyst

    b. spermatocele

    c. ascites

    d. hydrocele

14. A patient presents for a scrotal sonogram with a history of vasectomy and scrotal discomfort. Multiple cystic structures are seen in both testes along the mediastinum testis. Color Doppler does not demonstrate any flow in these cystic structures. What is the likely diagnosis?

    a. tubular ectasia of the rete testis

    b. bilateral spermatoceles

    c. simple intratesticular cysts

    d. bilateral seminoma

15. A 26-year-old man presents with fever, scrotal pain, and swelling. The sonogram shows an enlarged hypoechoic epididymis with hyperemia. A small hydrocele is noted. The testis appears normal. What is the likely diagnosis?

    a. orchitis

    b. epididymitis

    c. epididymo-orchitis

    d. testicular torsion

16. What is the most common correctable cause of male infertility?
    a. undescended testis
    b. spermatocele
    c. varicocele
    d. hydrocele

17. A 42-year-old patient presents with a painless right scrotal mass. Sonographically, a 2.5-cm, irregular, hypoechoic mass is seen in the mid-right testis. Color Doppler demonstrates hyperemia. The remainder of the scrotum, including the scrotal wall, appears normal. What is the most likely diagnosis?
    a. isolated orchitis
    b. testicular abscess
    c. seminoma
    d. intratesticular varicocele

18. A patient presents for a scrotal sonogram with a history of infertility. The testes appear normal bilaterally. Superior to the testes, multiple cystic structures are seen. The largest of these structures measures 4 mm. Color Doppler demonstrates flow within these structures and increased flow is seen when the patient is asked to perform the Valsalva maneuver. What is the likely diagnosis?
    a. spermatoceles
    b. epididymal cysts
    c. varicocele
    d. tubular ectasia of the rete testis

19. What is the most common sonographic appearance of a malignant testicular mass?
    a. hyperechoic with diffuse calcifications
    b. complex mass with thick septations
    c. cystic mass with ring calcifications
    d. hypoechoic mass

20. Which of the following lab values may be elevated with a testicular malignancy?
    a. PSA
    b. AFP
    c. ALP
    d. AST

Fill-in-the-Blank

1. Most intratesticular masses are considered _____ until proven otherwise, whereas the majority of extra-testicular masses are _____.

2. The major structures located within the scrotum are the _____, _____, and _____. The normal measurement of the scrotal wall is _____ in thickness. The _____ _____ divides the scrotum into two compartments.

3. The spermatic cord is composed of the _____ artery, _____ artery, and _____ artery; veins of the _____ _____, _____, _____, _____ _____; and connective tissue.

4. The head of the epididymis is located _____ to the testis and measures _____ in AP diameter. The head of the epididymis is best visualized in the _____ plane. The body and tail of the epididymis are usually _____ and _____ to the testis.

5. The primary function of the testes is the production of _____, which occurs in the _____ tubules, and _____, which is produced by the cells of _____.

6. The _____ _____ is a peritoneal sac composed of two layers, the _____ and _____ layers that cover and surround the testis and epididymis. The _____ layer covers the testis and the _____ layer is the inner lining of the scrotal wall.

7. The _____ _____ is seen sonographically as an echogenic band within the testis. It functions as a supporting system for arteries, veins, lymphatics, and seminiferous tubules.

8. The normal adult testis measures _____ in length and _____ in transverse and AP diameters.

9. Testicular torsion occurs when the _____ _____ twists. _____ drainage is affected first followed by _____ occlusion. Sonographic visualization of a _____ _____ is the most specific sign of testicular torsion.

10. Torsion of the _____ _____ and _____ _____ can cause acute scrotal pain mimicking testicular torsion.

11. Inflammation of the epididymis is called _____, whereas inflammation of the testis is called _____. On color Doppler affected or inflamed areas will demonstrate _____.

12. The most common cause of painless scrotal swelling is _____. Acquired hydroceles are associated with _____, _____, _____, or trauma.

13. An acute hydrocele will typically displace the testis in the _____ direction. Echogenic inflammatory deposits that are located on the tunica vaginalis are called _____ _____.

14. The most common epididymal lesions are _____ and _____ _____. _____ are located in the head of the epididymis, whereas _____ _____ can be located throughout the epididymis.

15. A varicocele is formed by a dilatation of the veins of the _____ _____. Veins greater than _____ are considered dilated. The majority of varicoceles occur on the _____ side. Having the patient perform the _____ maneuver can aid in the diagnosis by demonstrating an increase in flow.

16. Scrotal hernias typically contain _____ or _____ that has protruded through a patent processus _____.

17. An accumulation of blood located between the layers of the tunica vaginalis is called a _____ and is usually the result of _____, _____, _____, or _____.

18. The majority of intratesticular tumors are malignant. Benign intratesticular tumors are rare, but do occur and include _____ cell tumors and _____ cell tumors.

19. Intratubular testicular calcifications are called _____ and can be diagnosed if more than _____ echogenic foci are seen per transducer field. This condition warrants follow-up sonography because it has been associated with _____ _____.

20. The most common testicular malignancy is the _____, which is a _____ cell tumor. The second most common malignancy is the _____ cell carcinoma, which is commonly associated with elevated _____ and _____ levels.

Short Answer

1. Discuss the common indications for scrotal sonography.

2. When evaluating a patient with acute scrotal pain, it has been suggested that the sonographer should always evaluate the asymptomatic side first. Why is this true? Why are comparison images important?

3. Describe the clinical presentation, the most common sonographic appearance, and associated findings in a patient with a seminoma.

4. The diagnosis of an undescended testis is important because this condition can lead to more serious complications later in life. What conditions are associated with cryptorchidism?

5. Describe the sonographic appearance and associated findings seen with epididymo-orchitis.

IMAGE EVALUATION/PATHOLOGY

Review the images and answer the following questions.

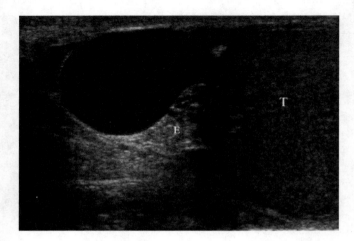

1. A 38-year-old patient presents with a painless, palpable lump in the superior aspect of the scrotum. Describe what is seen in this image. Give two possible diagnoses.

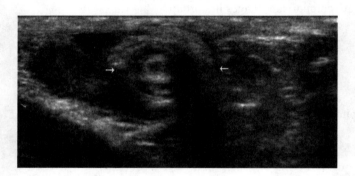

2. A 15-year-old patient presents with acute scrotal pain, nausea, and vomiting. The patient is extremely tender during the examination. This image is taken superior to the epididymis and testis in the region of the spermatic cord. What is seen in this image, indicated by the *arrow*, and what is this indicative of?

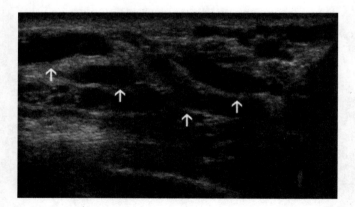

3. This patient presents with a palpable lump that corresponds sonographically to an epididymal cyst. This image is taken superior to the testis and epididymis on the left side. What do the *arrows* represent? What is the normal measurement of these structures? What would you do next to confirm your diagnosis?

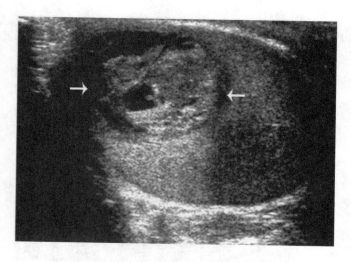

4. Describe the mass seen in this image. Which testicular tumors are more likely to have this appearance?

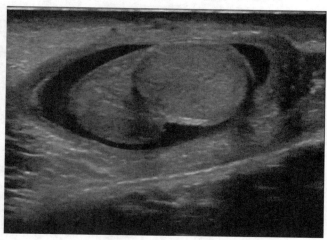

5. A 30-year-old patient presents with acute scrotal pain, an enlarged scrotum, and fever. Describe everything that is seen in this image. Hypervascularity of the epididymis was also noted. Flow in the testis was normal. What is the diagnosis?

CASE STUDIES

Review the images and answer the following questions.

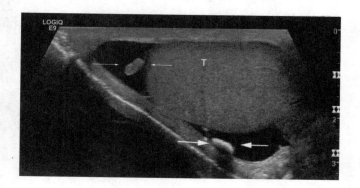

1. A 50-year-old man presents with painless scrotal enlargement on the left side. What structure is identified by the *small arrows*? What does the structure indicated by the *large arrows* represent? What can cause this? What other pathology is seen? Can this pathology cause any other concerns?

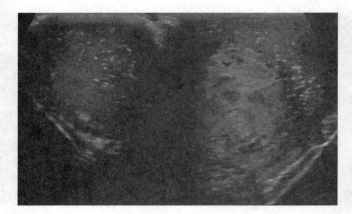

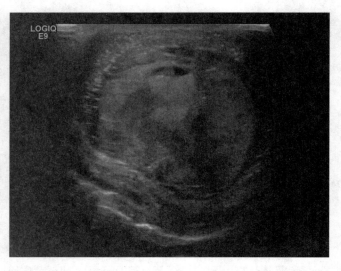

2. These images were taken in a 45-year-old man who presented with a large, firm, left testicular lump. Describe what is seen in these two images. What is the likely diagnosis?

The Musculoskeletal System

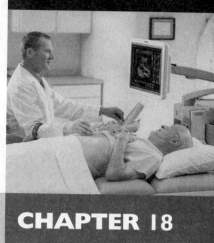

REVIEW OF GLOSSARY TERMS

Matching

Match the terms with their definitions.

KEY TERMS

1. _____ amphiarthrosis

2. _____ anisotropy

3. _____ diarthrosis

4. _____ endomysium

5. _____ enthesis

6. _____ epimysium

7. _____ fascicle

8. _____ paratenon

9. _____ perimysium

10. _____ retinaculum

DEFINITION

a. Small bundle or cluster of fibers
b. Properties vary with direction
c. Joint permitting little motion, such as vertebrae
d. Connective tissue surrounds an individual muscle fiber
e. General term for a band or band-like structure binding organs or tissue to hold them together
f. Joint permitting free motion, such as the shoulder
g. Site of attachment of a muscle or ligament to bone
h. Connective tissue surrounds a bundle of muscle fiber
i. Fatty areolar tissue filling the interstices of the facial compartment in which a tendon is situated
j. Connective tissue surrounds entire muscle

ANATOMY AND PHYSIOLOGY REVIEW

Image Labeling

Complete the labels in the images that follow.

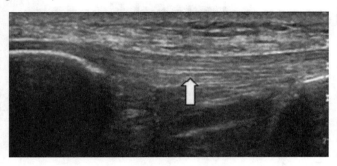

1. What type of structure is identified by the *white arrow*?

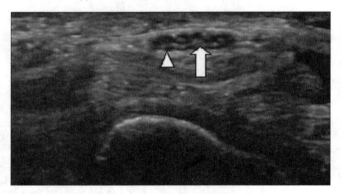

2. What type of structure is identified by the large *white arrow*?

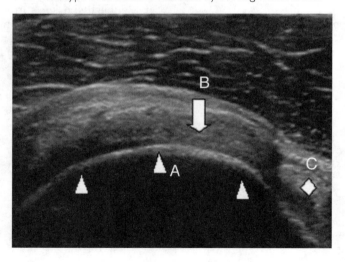

3. Shoulder anatomy

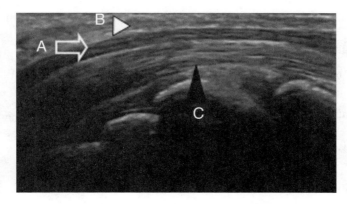

4. Carpal tunnel anatomy

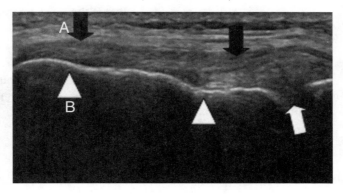

5. Anatomy of the medial knee

CHAPTER REVIEW

Multiple Choice

Complete each question by circling the best answer.

1. Which of the following is a major benefit of using sonography to evaluate the musculoskeletal system?
   a. Spermatic always accedes the accuracy of MRI.
   b. Sonography uses less ionizing radiation than CT.
   c. Sonography is easy to learn.
   d. Sonography is a dynamic examination.

2. Which of the following planes are commonly used when imaging the musculoskeletal system?
   a. sagittal and transverse
   b. radial and antiradial
   c. long axis and short axis
   d. scan planes are not described when imaging the MSK system

3. What attaches bone to muscle?
   a. fibrocartilage
   b. tendons
   c. nerves
   d. ligaments

4. Which of the following structures is NOT contained in a neurovascular bundle?
   a. artery
   b. vein
   c. tendon
   d. nerves

5. Which of the following attaches bone to bone, providing needed stability and strength?
   a. fibrocartilage
   b. tendons
   c. nerves
   d. ligaments

6. Which of the following is NOT evaluated in a shoulder examination for rotator cuff injury?
   a. biceps tendon
   b. triceps tendon
   c. supraspinatus tendon
   d. infraspinatus tendon

7. Which of the following statements regarding the acromioclavicular joint is FALSE?

   a. Abnormal fluid collections may form here in cases of supraspinatus tendon pathology.

   b. The joint space is wedge-shaped from posterior to anterior.

   c. The AC joint is a common site for arthritis and osteophytes.

   d. The AC joint is best evaluated in external rotation.

8. Which of the following shares a common insertion point with the supraspinatus tendon on the greater tuberosity of the humerus?

   a. infraspinatus tendon

   b. biceps tendon

   c. subscapularis tendon

   d. triceps tendon

9. When evaluating the shoulder with sonography, which of the following is NOT considered a major rotator cuff pathology?

   a. cuff atrophy

   b. absence of cuff

   c. abnormal fluid collection

   d. hyperechoic defect

10. Which of the following structures is NOT found in the anterior elbow?

    a. median nerve

    b. ulnar nerve

    c. brachial artery

    d. distal biceps tendon

11. What is the term for tennis elbow?

    a. common flexor osteotendinopathy

    b. biceps osteotendinopathy

    c. common extensor tendinopathy

    d. olecranon bursitis

12. Which of the following is NOT found on the palmar wrist?

    a. flexor tendons

    b. EPB and APL

    c. median nerve

    d. ulnar and radial nerves

13. Carpal tunnel syndrome results from compression of what nerve?

    a. ulnar nerve

    b. radial nerve

    c. palmar nerve

    d. median nerve

14. What is the most common pathology of the knee?

    a. rupture of the MCL

    b. Baker cyst

    c. quadriceps tendon rupture

    d. torn meniscus

15. What is the most frequently injured joint in the body?

    a. Knee

    b. Shoulder

    c. Ankle

    d. Hip

16. What is the most commonly affected anatomic structure of the posterior ankle?

    a. Achilles tendon

    b. plantaris tendon

    c. posterior tibialis tendon

    d. flexor digitorum tendon

17. How many tarsal bones make up the foot?

    a. three

    b. five

    c. seven

    d. nine

18. Which section of the plantar fascia is most commonly affected in plantar fasciitis?

    a. medial

    b. central

    c. lateral

    d. posterior

19. What is the most commonly injured ankle ligament?

    a. tibiofibular ligament

    b. calcaneal fibular ligament

    c. anterior talofibular ligament

    d. peroneus longus ligament

20. Which of the following describes the function of the plantar fascia?

    a. arch support

    b. gait

    c. distribution of weight

    d. all of the above are functions of the plantar fascia

Fill-in-the-Blank

1. _____ refers to the change in the properties of a structure when measured or evaluated in different directions.

2. A technique called _____ _____ involves using an abundance of gel to avoid using excessive pressure when evaluating superficial structures.

3. A _____ is a collection of loose connective tissue between the sheath and tendon that aids in tendon movement.

4. A _____ is a synovial lined pouch that produces viscous fluid that aides in tendon or muscle slip.

5. When imaged in the short axis, the nerve has a _____ pattern, with the _____ nerve fibers surrounded by the _____ perineuron or connective tissue.

6. _____ is found in the meniscus and intervertebral disk spaces and acts as a shock absorber. _____ or _____ cartilage lies at the terminal ends of bone in any joint.

7. The biceps tendon is a _____ of the forearm and _____ of the elbow and shoulder.

8. The supraspinatus tendon is an _____ of the humerus and also provides stabilization of the _____ _____ in the glenohumeral joint.

9. The radial fossa and coronoid fossa can be evaluated with sonography for joint effusions. Excessive fluid in the joint results in the fat pads being displaced _____ away from the bone.

10. The primary function of the triceps is _____ of the elbow.

11. Common flexor osteotendinopathy refers to pathology of the _____ _____ tendons and the _____ _____ at insertion. This is also called _____ _____.

12. The most commonly affected section in common extensor tendinopathy is the _____ _____ _____ _____ _____. The transducer is typically placed on top of the _____ _____ in the _____ plane to start the evaluation.

13. The distal biceps tendon inserts _____ on the _____ _____ of the radius. Pathology can include _____ or _____ thickness tears.

14. On the volar aspect of the wrist are the _____ tendons and _____, _____ and _____ nerve. The most commonly evaluated area on the volar wrist is the _____ _____.

15. The quadriceps tendon is an important _____ of the lower extremity. Over 95% of the fibers of the quadriceps tendon insert on the _____ _____.

16. The _____ _____ is the primary ligamentous support structure for the medial knee. The _____ tears generally occur from the joint space, whereas the _____ tears can occur anywhere along the length of the tendon.

17. Evaluation of the posterior knee typically focuses on the _____ _____, more commonly known as the _____ _____. This typically presents as a palpable mass in the _____ _____.

18. The _____ aspect of the ankle is the most often injured area of the ankle due to _____ foot injuries.

19. The tendons of the medial ankle are the PTT or _____ _____ _____. Directly posterior is the FDL or _____ _____ _____, the most posterior is the FHL or _____ _____ _____.

20. The longest and strongest tendon of the body is the _____. The _____ _____ area is the most common site for rupture. This is _____ proximal to the insertion on the calcaneus.

Short Answer

1. Describe the sonographic appearance of a normal tendon.

2. When imaging a tendon, why is it important to be perpendicular to the structure?

3. Describe the normal sonographic appearance of nerves.

4. List the major criteria used to diagnose rotator cuff pathology. What are the minor criteria?

5. What anatomical landmarks are used to evaluate the popliteal fossa for a Baker cyst? What diagnostic criteria are used to ensure a Baker cyst is the correct diagnosis?

IMAGE EVALUATION/PATHOLOGY

Review the images and answer the following questions.

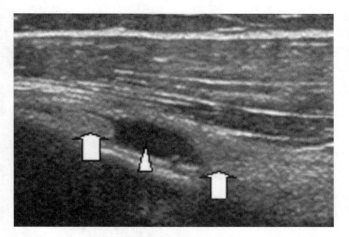

1. In this image, the *white arrows* represent the biceps tendon. What does the anechoic space indicated by the *white arrowhead* represent? What pathology is seen here?

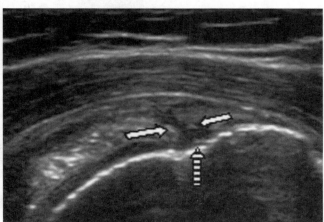

2. In this image of the shoulder, what is represented by the *white arrows*?

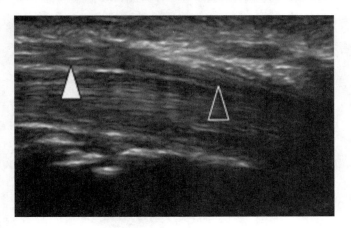

3. Explain what pathology is present in this image of the median nerve at the proximal carpal tunnel.

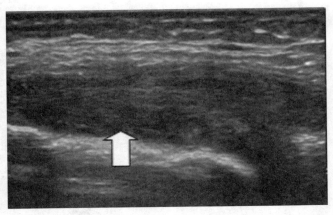

4. This image was taken over the medial knee. Describe what is seen in this medial collateral ligament.

5. This patient presents with pain in the posterior knee. What pathology is seen here?

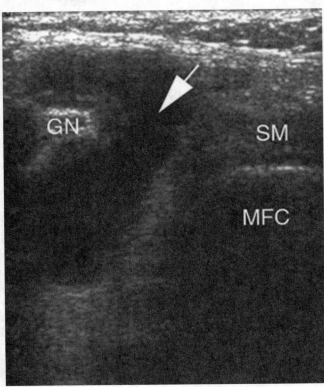

CASE STUDY

Review the images and answer the following questions.

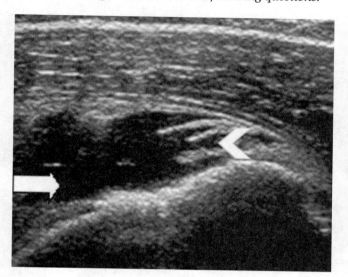 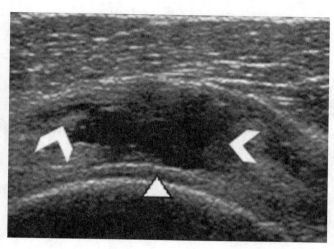

1. This 47-year-old man presents with increasing shoulder pain and an inability to lift his arm over his head. Describe the pathology seen in these images. What is the diagnosis?

PART 3

NEONATAL AND PEDIATRIC SONOGRAPHY

The Pediatric Abdomen

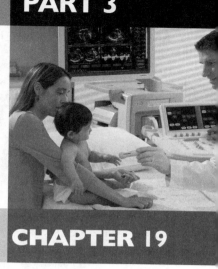

REVIEW OF GLOSSARY TERMS

Matching

Match the terms with their definitions.

KEY TERMS

1. _____ AFP

2. _____ biloma

3. _____ coarctation

4. _____ hemobilia

5. _____ hemoperitoneum

6. _____ hyperalimentation

7. _____ hyponatremia

8. _____ ileus

9. _____ jaundice

DEFINITION

a. The administration of nutrients through IV feeding
b. A narrowing or constriction
c. A tumor marker frequently elevated in cases of hepatocellular carcinoma, hepatoblastoma, and certain testicular cancers
d. Yellowish pigmentation of the skin and whites of the eyes caused by increased levels of bilirubin
e. A walled-off collection of bile caused by a disruption of the biliary tree
f. Failure of the normal propulsion of the digestive tract
g. Blood in the peritoneal cavity
h. Hemorrhage or blood in the bile caused by bleeding into the biliary tree
i. An electrolyte imbalance; low sodium levels in the blood

ANATOMY AND PHYSIOLOGY REVIEW

Image Labeling

Complete the labels in the images that follow.

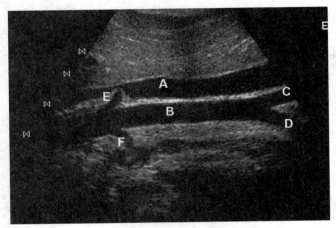

1. Abdominal vasculature

CHAPTER REVIEW

Multiple Choice

Complete each question by circling the best answer.

1. Which of the following statements regarding hemangioendothelioma is FALSE?
   a. Infants less than 6 months of age are typically affected.
   b. Patients are typically asymptomatic.
   c. The lesions may be hypoechoic or hyperechoic.
   d. The lesions may rupture causing hemoperitoneum.

2. Which of the following pediatric liver tumors is malignant?
   a. mesenchymal hamartoma
   b. cavernous hemangioma
   c. hepatoblastoma
   d. hemangioendothelioma

3. Which type of hepatitis most often affects children and young adults?
   a. hepatitis A
   b. hepatitis B
   c. hepatitis C
   d. hepatitis D

4. A pediatric patient presents with a history of fatty infiltration. Which of the following causes of fatty infiltration of the liver is irreversible?
   a. obesity
   b. diabetes mellitus
   c. hepatitis A
   d. Reye syndrome

5. In infants and children, which of the following may cause cirrhosis of the liver?
   a. biliary atresia
   b. cystic fibrosis
   c. metabolic diseases
   d. all of the above may cause cirrhosis

6. Which of the following describes the most common sonographic appearance of a cirrhotic liver?
   a. enlarged, hypoechoic liver with echogenic portal triads
   b. small, hyperechoic liver with a heterogeneous echotexture
   c. small, hypoechoic liver with cystic spaces seen throughout the parenchyma
   d. enlarged, hyperechoic liver with a smooth contour and homogeneous echotexture

7. Which of the following is a rare liver condition that is associated with autosomal recessive polycystic disease?

   a. fulminant hepatitis

   b. hemosiderosis

   c. hepatic fibrosis

   d. hemangioendothelioma

8. Which of the following is NOT a primary malignant liver tumor?

   a. hepatoblastoma

   b. hepatoma

   c. hemangioendothelioma

   d. embryonal sarcoma

9. Which of the following laboratory values is usually elevated with a primary pediatric hepatic malignancy?

   a. PSA

   b. Beta-hCG

   c. CA-125

   d. AFP

10. What is the most common pediatric liver mass?

    a. cavernous hemangioma

    b. hepatoblastoma

    c. mesenchymal hamartoma

    d. hepatoma

11. Which disease results in the absence of the intrahepatic and extrahepatic ducts near the porta hepatis and possibly the absence of the gallbladder?

    a. choledochal cyst

    b. Caroli disease

    c. sclerosing cholangitis

    d. biliary atresia

12. An infant presents with a palpable abdominal mass and jaundice. Sonographically, a large cystic mass is seen near the porta hepatis. A normal gallbladder is also visualized separate from the cystic mass. What is the most likely diagnosis?

    a. choledochal cyst

    b. Caroli disease

    c. sclerosing cholangitis

    d. biliary atresia

13. During your abdominal evaluation on a pediatric patient, you notice the gallbladder is small even though the patient has been fasting. Which of the following is NOT a cause of a small or nondistended gallbladder?

    a. viral hepatitis

    b. cystic fibrosis

    c. obstruction of the common bile duct

    d. congenital hypoplasia

14. Gallstones are not as commonly seen in the pediatric population; however, certain conditions predispose an infant or child to developing gallstones. Which of the following conditions does NOT predispose a patient to gallstones?

    a. sickle cell disease

    b. cystic fibrosis

    c. hemolytic anemia

    d. pancreatitis

15. A 1-month-old boy presents with projectile vomiting and symptoms of dehydration. An olive-shaped mass can be palpated in the epigastric region. What pathology are you looking for as you evaluate the abdomen in this patient?

    a. hypertrophic pyloric stenosis

    b. choledochal cyst

    c. biliary atresia

    d. annular pancreas

16. Which of the following statements regarding hypertrophic pyloric stenosis is FALSE?

    a. The stomach is often filled with fluid, even if the patient has been fasting.

    b. Sonographically, a donut sign is seen with a hyperechoic central lumen surrounded by a hypoechoic muscle.

    c. The stomach wall is also grossly enlarged with hypertrophic pyloric stenosis.

    d. The pylorus is considered abnormal when the length from the antrum to the distal end exceeds 1.8 cm.

17. Duodenal atresia is common in patients with which of the following?

    a. trisomy 13

    b. trisomy 15

    c. trisomy 18

    d. trisomy 21

18. An infant presents with a history of vomiting. While evaluating the patient, you notice a vessel immediately anterior to the SMA. With further evaluation, this vessel is identified as the SMV. What condition is associated with this finding?

    a. midgut malrotation

    b. suodenal atresia

    c. rhabdomyosarcoma

    d. intussusception

19. The most common obstructive bowel disorder of early childhood occurs when a segment of bowel prolapses into a more distal segment and is called what?

    a. midgut malrotation

    b. duodenal atresia

    c. rhabdomyosarcoma

    d. intussusception

20. An 8-year-old patient presents with right lower quadrant pain, nausea, and fever. An 8-mm, non-compressible structure with a target appearance in the transverse axis is visualized in the right lower quadrant. With color Doppler, hyperemia of the structure is noted. What is the most likely diagnosis?
    a. Crohn disease
    b. appendicitis
    c. midgut malrotation
    d. intussusception

Fill-in-the-Blank

1. Patient preparation for an abdominal sonogram in a pediatric patient will vary depending on the age of the patient. Infants are fed every _____; therefore, the examination should be scheduled just before a feeding. Children 1 to 3 years of age should fast for _____, and older children should fast for _____.

2. The IVC may be interrupted and drain via an _____ continuation. The hemiazygous continuation lies more _____ to the aorta.

3. Cavernous hemangiomas are more common in _____ and usually become evident around _____ of age. The typical sonographic appearance is a well-defined, _____ mass.

4. The symptoms of acute viral hepatitis are similar to those of _____ _____. One difference is that the _____ is usually larger in _____ than in acute viral hepatitis.

5. A liver abscess in infants is usually the result of an infection from the _____ or _____ and usually enters the liver through a contaminated _____ or _____ vein.

6. Primary liver tumors are _____ common in children than in adults and _____ of all pediatric hepatic tumors are malignant.

7. Vessel involvement generally indicates _____ hepatic disease rather than hepatic _____. The most common clinical signs of hepatoblastoma are _____ and painless _____ abdominal mass.

8. Differential diagnosis for a hepatoblastoma include _____, _____ _____, and _____ _____.

9. Metastatic hepatic lesions are frequently associated with _____ _____, _____, _____, and _____.

10. Conjugated hyperbilirubinemia in a newborn may be caused by diseases of the _____, such as _____, or _____ _____ abnormalities, such as _____ _____.

11. Biliary atresia presents clinically as persistent neonatal _____ at _____ of age. Symptoms are similar to neonatal _____ and neonatal _____.

12. Children with _____ _____ _____ and _____ _____ are pre-disposed to the formation of sludge and gallstones.

13. An inflammatory fibrosis that obliterates the intra and extrahepatic bile ducts is called _____ _____, and the majority of children with this condition have associated inflammatory _____ disease.

14. A solid, malignant tumor that arises in the biliary tract in children is _____. It is the second most common cause of _____ _____ in older children.

15. Cystic fibrosis affects the _____ glands in the _____ and _____ tract. In patients with cystic fibrosis, the pancreas is _____ due to the replacement of pancreatic tissue by fibrosis and fatty tissue.

16. In patients with pyloric stenosis, the AP diameter of the pylorus exceeds _____, the length of the antrum to the distal end of the channel exceeds _____, and the muscle thickness exceeds _____.

17. Duodenal atresia is an _____ cause of a dilated duodenum and stomach. Extrinsic causes of an obstruction at this level include _____, _____ _____ cyst, _____ cyst, and _____ pancreas.

18. With midgut malrotation the relationship of the following vessels should be evaluated: the _____ and _____. If volvulus is present, the _____ _____ on gray scale and color Doppler has high sensitivity and specificity for the disorder.

19. The most common type of intussusception is _____ and presents with _____ _____, _____ _____ stool, and a palpable _____ _____. Most occur between the ages of _____ _____.

20. Bowel diseases such as Crohn disease and intussusception typically have a _____ or _____ appearance in the transverse axis and may have a _____ appearance in the longitudinal axis.

Short Answer

1. While scanning a pediatric patient, a hyperechoic solid liver tumor is noted. List the differential diagnoses for a solid, hyperechoic liver tumor in a pediatric patient.

2. List the causes of fatty infiltration of the liver in the pediatric population.

3. Describe the common sonographic appearance of a primary liver malignancy in the pediatric patient. What other surrounding structures must be evaluated when a liver tumor is diagnosed?

4. Hepatoblastoma is associated with a number of other conditions. List the conditions that increase a child's risk of developing a hepatoblastoma. At what age does this tumor typically occur?

5. You are asked to perform an abdominal sonogram on a pediatric patient with a history of cystic fibrosis. What abdominal pathology might you expect to find in a patient with this diagnosis?

IMAGE EVALUATION/PATHOLOGY

Review the images and answer the following questions.

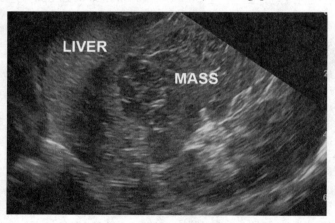

1. This 3-month-old patient presents with a palpable abdominal mass. Describe the mass seen in this image. List the differential diagnoses for this mass.

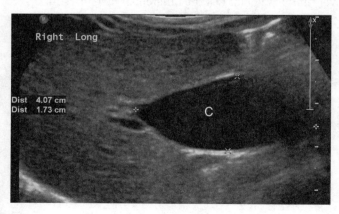

2. A 4-month-old patient presents with a palpable right upper quadrant mass and jaundice. This cystic structure is seen within the porta hepatis. The gallbladder is separate from the cystic structure and appears normal. What is the likely diagnosis?

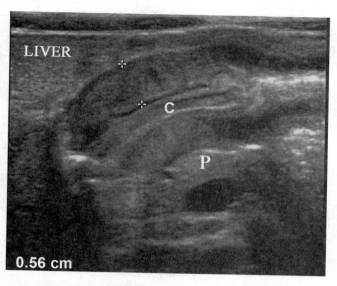

3. A 1-month-old boy presents with a history of projectile vomiting and weight loss. This image was taken in the epigastric region. What is seen in this image? What does the P represent? What measurements will help confirm the diagnosis?

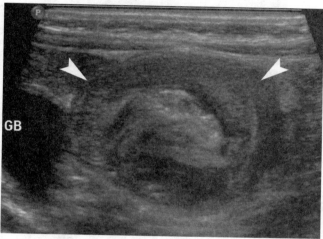

4. A 1-year-old patient presents with pain and a palpable mass in the right upper quadrant. This image was taken over the palpable mass. What is the most likely diagnosis of a lesion in the bowel that presents with this target sign pattern?

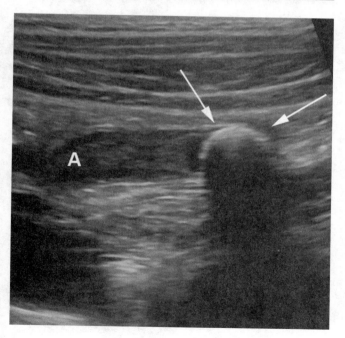

5. This 7-year-old patient presents with severe right lower quadrant pain with fever, nausea, and vomiting. What is seen in this image of the right lower quadrant? What are the *arrows* pointing to?

CASE STUDIES

Review the images and answer the following questions.

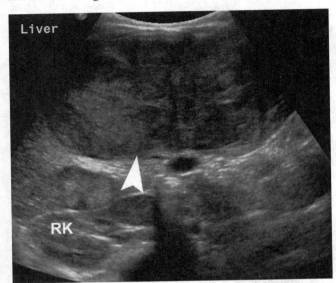

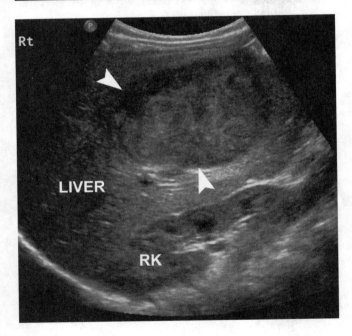

1. A 4-year-old patient presents with a palpable abdominal mass. These images are taken from the right lobe of the liver. Describe what is seen. What is the most likely diagnosis? What lab value is typically elevated with this pathology? What other structures should be evaluated for involvement?

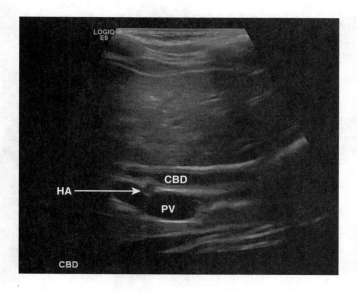

2. An 8-year-old patient presents with right upper quadrant pain and jaundice. This image of the porta hepatis demonstrates thickening of the walls of the common bile duct. What pathology could cause this? What associated condition is typically found concurrent with this pathology?

The Pediatric Urinary System and Adrenal Glands

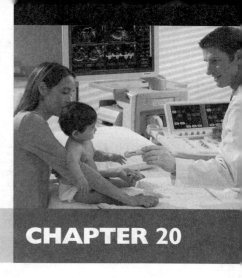

REVIEW OF GLOSSARY TERMS

Matching

Match the terms with their definitions.

KEY TERMS

1. _____ diuresis

2. _____ enuresis

3. _____ hydronephrosis

4. _____ reflux

5. _____ ureteropelvic junction

6. _____ ureterovesical junction

DEFINITION

a. Occurs when valves at the junction of the ureter and bladder allow urine from the bladder to back up into the ureter and kidney
b. Involuntary discharge of urine during sleep
c. Dilatation of the collecting system of the urinary tract
d. Area where the ureter enters into the urinary bladder
e. Increased secretion or production of urine
f. Area where the renal pelvis connects to the ureter

ANATOMY AND PHYSIOLOGY REVIEW

Image Labeling

Complete the labels in the images that follow.

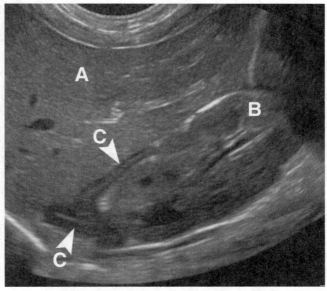

1. Normal sonographic anatomy

CHAPTER REVIEW

Multiple Choice

Complete each question by circling the best answer.

1. Which of the following normal structures may be mistaken for a renal cyst in infants and young children?
   a. renal cortex
   b. renal pyramids
   c. column of Bertin
   d. fetal lobulation

2. Which of the following is a normal finding in a neonate?
   a. bilateral echogenic kidneys with prominent pyramids
   b. bilateral hypoechoic kidneys with hyperechoic renal sinus
   c. echogenic kidneys with a dilated renal pelvis measuring 2 cm
   d. bilateral kidneys isoechoic to the liver with prominent hyperechoic renal pyramids

3. Which pathology demonstrates echogenic renal pyramids resulting from calcium deposits?
   a. medullary sponge kidney
   b. leukemia
   c. renal artery stenosis
   d. chronic renal infections

4. What should the normal resistive indices in the interlobar and arcuate arteries of a pediatric patient be?
   a. greater than 0.7
   b. less than 0.7
   c. greater than 0.5
   d. less than 0.5

5. Which of the following statements is FALSE in cases of bilateral renal agenesis?
   a. Bilateral renal agenesis may be detected during an obstetric sonogram.
   b. Bilateral renal agenesis is associated with Potter's syndrome.
   c. An overly distended urinary bladder is common in cases of bilateral renal agenesis.
   d. The adrenal glands may lie in the renal fossa and be mistaken for kidneys in cases of bilateral renal agenesis.

6. What is the most frequent site of urinary obstruction in infants?
   a. the ureterovesical junction
   b. the distal urethra
   c. the ureteropelvic junction
   d. the distal ureter

7. What is the most common cause of urethral obstruction in boys?
   a. enlarged prostate
   b. ureterocele
   c. posterior urethral valves
   d. neurogenic bladder

8. Which of the following is seen with posterior urethral valves?
   a. unilateral hydronephrosis seen in utero
   b. thickening of the renal cortex
   c. enlarged, thin-walled bladder
   d. dilated tortuous ureters

9. Prune belly syndrome is NOT associated with which pathological finding?
   a. cryptorchidism
   b. dysplastic kidneys
   c. Wilm tumor
   d. absent abdominal muscles

10. A neonate presents with a history of suspected renal abnormality diagnosed during a prenatal sonogram. On the current sonogram, both kidneys appear symmetrically enlarged and diffusely echogenic. A differentiation between the renal sinus, medulla, and cortex is not seen. What is the most likely diagnosis?
    a. Prune belly syndrome
    b. bilateral renal hypoplasia
    c. medullary sponge kidney
    d. infantile polycystic kidney disease

11. A male neonate presents with a history of suspected renal abnormality seen on a prenatal sonogram. On examination, the right kidney is normal; however, the left kidney appears to be composed of multiple cysts of varying sizes. No normal renal parenchyma or sinus is visualized. The bladder is also normal. What is the most likely diagnosis?
    a. unilateral renal agenesis
    b. multicystic dysplastic kidney
    c. hypoplasia of the left kidney
    d. infantile polycystic kidney disease

12. An infant presents with a palpable mass just inferior to the umbilicus. The area appears red and inflamed. Sonography reveals a cystic area located between the umbilicus and the urinary bladder. What is the most likely diagnosis?

    a. bladder diverticulum

    b. urachal cyst

    c. multicystic dysplastic kidney

    d. umbilical hernia

13. What is infantile polycystic kidney disease associated with?

    a. medullary sponge kidney

    b. congenital hepatic fibrosis

    c. multicystic dysplastic kidney

    d. tuberous sclerosis

14. What is the most common malignant renal tumor in the pediatric population?

    a. Wilm tumor

    b. neuroblastoma

    c. renal cell carcinoma

    d. mesoblastic nephroma

15. A 3-year-old presents with a palpable right sided flank mass. Sonographically, a large, homogeneous, well-circumscribed mass is seen extending from the superior pole of the right kidney. A few cystic spaces are noted within the lesion. What is the most likely diagnosis?

    a. mesoblastic nephroma

    b. renal cell carcinoma

    c. Wilm tumor

    d. angiomyolipoma

16. A neonate is born with a palpable left flank mass. Sonography reveals a large solid homogeneous mass in the left kidney. Very little normal renal parenchyma is seen. What is the most likely diagnosis in this age group?

    a. mesoblastic nephroma

    b. renal cell carcinoma

    c. Wilm tumor

    d. angiomyolipoma

17. A 2-month-old infant presents with an enlarging, palpable left flank mass and mild hypertension. Sonographically, a large, solid, ill-defined echogenic mass is seen superior to the left kidney. Calcifications with shadowing are present within the mass. The kidney appears to be displaced inferiorly. What is the most likely diagnosis?

    a. Wilm tumor

    b. adrenal hemorrhage

    c. neuroblastoma

    d. adrenal metastasis

18. What is the most common children adrenal tumor?

    a. Wilm tumor

    b. pheochromocytoma

    c. neuroblastoma

    d. nephroblastoma

19. Which of the following statements regarding adrenal hemorrhage is FALSE?

    a. Adrenal hemorrhage is typically diagnosed when the infant is 1 month old.

    b. Infants who are premature or have neonatal sepsis, hypoxia, and birth trauma may develop an adrenal hemorrhage.

    c. Jaundice may occur, as well as scrotal discoloration in male infants.

    d. Blunt abdominal trauma or child abuse may cause hemorrhage in older infants.

20. Which statement regarding the location of the adrenal glands is TRUE?

    a. The adrenal glands are located within the anterior pararenal space.

    b. The right adrenal gland lies between the right crus of the diaphragm and the liver, posterior to the IVC.

    c. The left adrenal gland is medial and to the right of the left crus of the diaphragm and anterior to the pancreatic tail.

    d. With renal agenesis, the adrenal glands are typically harder to locate.

Fill-in-the-Blank

1. Renal _____ are seen as an irregular renal outline and are commonly seen in _____ but should disappear by about _____ of age.

2. The cortical echogenicity of the kidneys in neonates and infants, particularly _____ infants, is _____ than that in older children.

3. The normal renal artery in a pediatric patient should demonstrate a sharp _____ peak with continuous forward _____ flow.

4. The resistive indices can help determine if a dilated urinary system is _____. The RI is increased in _____ disease and _____ disease.

5. Bilateral renal agenesis is associated with _____, or a decrease in amniotic fluid, _____ syndrome, and _____ hypoplasia.

6. A dilation of the collecting system, specifically the renal calyces, the renal pelvis, and ureters is called _____. The three most common causes are _____ obstruction, _____ _____ obstruction, and _____ _____ _____.

7. With hydronephrosis there should be recognizable renal _____ surrounding the dilated collecting system. In cases of bilateral hydronephrosis, the obstruction is going to be located _____ in the _____ or _____.

8. In patients with prune belly syndrome, the bladder is _____ and _____, whereas in a patient with posterior urethral valves the bladder is _____-walled.

9. A _____ _____ _____ develops from complete ureteral obstruction in utero. If the condition is _____, it is inconsistent with life.

10. Renal hypoplasia is a _____ but otherwise normal kidney and most often results from atrophy secondary to _____ or from _____ occlusion.

11. Tuberous sclerosis can present with bilateral renal _____ and _____.

12. Wilm tumor typically presents as a _____ _____ but may also present with _____, _____, _____, and _____ _____ _____ _____.

13. The peak age for a Wilm tumor is _____ years. Wilm tumor may be _____ and may invade the _____ vein and _____.

14. A cystic renal mass that appears as multiple thin-walled cysts or a large cyst with septations is called _____ _____ _____.

15. The most common sonographic finding in cases of pyelonephritis is _____ of the kidneys. Areas of _____ or, less often, _____ echogenicity may also be seen.

16. A solid bladder tumor that can occur in the pediatric population and may cause hematuria, dysuria, retention, and UTI is called _____.

17. A neuroblastoma typically occurs in _____ and rarely after the age of _____. They tend to have _____-defined borders and _____ are common.

18. A rare functioning adrenal tumor that originates in the chromaffin tissue is called _____. Common clinical symptoms include _____, _____, _____, and _____.

19. The adrenal glands are susceptible to hemorrhage due to their _____ _____ and high _____. Adrenal hemorrhage is most commonly identified between the _____ _____ _____ of life.

20. Adrenal abscess are the result of neonatal _____ and are usually _____. Clinical symptoms include _____, _____, and _____ _____.

Short Answer

1. Describe the differences in the sonographic appearance of the kidneys in infants, children, and adults.

2. Describe how hydronephrosis and multicystic dysplastic kidney can be distinguished sonographically.

3. When evaluating an abdominal mass, the sonographer must determine three important factors to make an accurate diagnosis. Describe the three factors.

4. Describe how a Wilm tumor would be differentiated from a neuroblastoma sonographically.

5. Describe how a neuroblastoma would be differentiated from an adrenal hemorrhage sonographically.

IMAGE EVALUATION/PATHOLOGY

Review the images and answer the following questions.

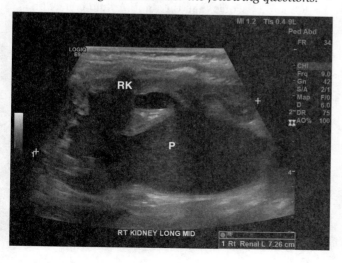

1. What pathology is seen in this image of the right kidney? What are the most common causes of this pathology in infants and children?

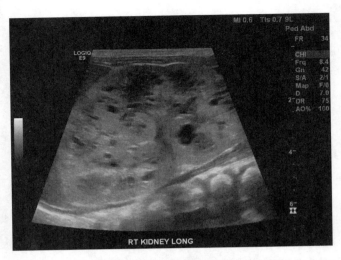

2. What pathology is seen in this image of the right kidney in a neonate? What liver condition is associated with this renal pathology?

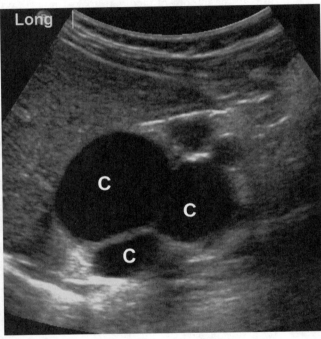

3. A 2-week-old infant presents for a renal sonogram to follow up an abnormality seen on a prenatal sonogram. This image was taken in the right upper quadrant. The left kidney and bladder appear normal. What is the likely diagnosis?

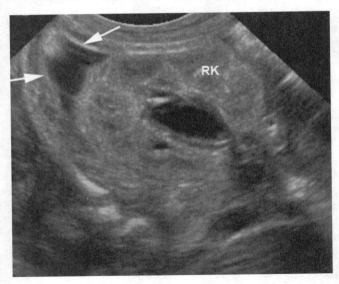

4. A male neonate presents with posterior urethral valves. Bilateral hydronephrosis is seen, with the left kidney worse than the right. A fluid collection is seen surrounding the right kidney, indicated by the *arrows* in this image. What does the fluid most likely represent?

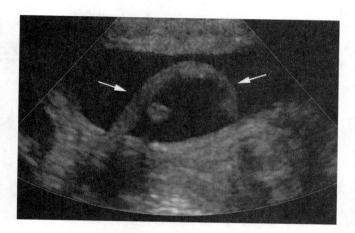

5. An infant presents for a renal sonogram. A duplicated collecting system is seen in the right kidney. The left kidney appears normal. The upper pole collecting system on the right is dilated. This image was taken in the urinary bladder. What are the *arrows* pointing to?

CASE STUDIES

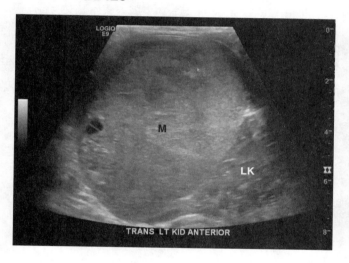

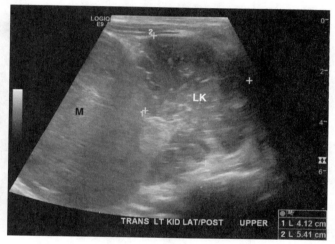

1. A 3-year-old boy presents with an enlarging palpable mass in the right upper quadrant. A large, solid mass is seen on the right kidney. Very little normal renal tissue is seen in the upper pole. Describe the mass. What is the most likely diagnosis? List the congenital malformations associated with this tumor.

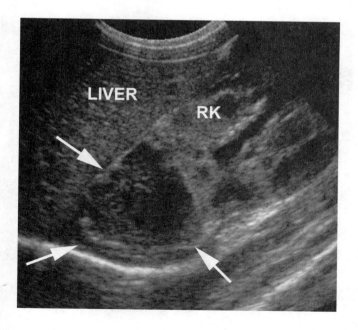

2. A 2-day-old premature newborn has clinical symptoms of anemia and jaundice. An abdominal sonogram is ordered. The only abnormal finding is a complex mass superior to the right kidney. What is the most likely diagnosis, given the patient's age and symptoms? How would you expect this mass to change if a follow-up sonogram is performed in a few weeks?

The Neonatal Brain

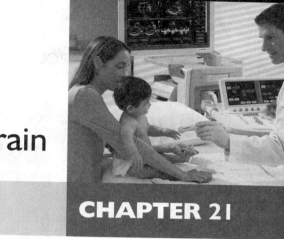

CHAPTER 21

REVIEW OF GLOSSARY TERMS

Matching

Match the terms with their definitions.

KEY TERMS

1. _____ cerebrum

2. _____ cerebellum

3. _____ choroid plexus

4. _____ Corpus callosum

5. _____ falx cerebri

6. _____ fontanelle

7. _____ hypoxia

8. _____ porencephaly

9. _____ thalamus

DEFINITION

a. Lack of oxygen

b. Echogenic cluster of cells located within the lateral ventricles responsible for the production of cerebral spinal fluid

c. Fold of dura matter that divides the two hemispheres of the brain

d. Largest section of the brain; divided into two hemispheres joined by the corpus callosum

e. Paired ovoid structures in the central brain responsible for relaying nerve impulses and carrying sensory information into the cerebral cortex

f. Posterior portion of the brain composed of two hemispheres

g. Cyst or cavity in the brain, usually the result of a destructive lesion

h. Soft spot between the cranial bones

i. Largest white matter structure in the brain; contains nerve tracts that allow communication between the right and left hemispheres of the brain

ANATOMY AND PHYSIOLOGY REVIEW

Image Labeling

Complete the labels in the images that follow.

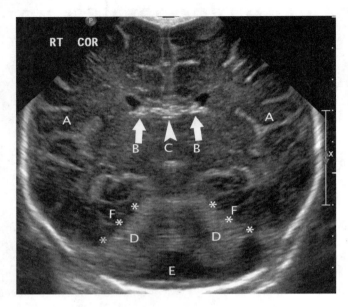

1. Coronal brain

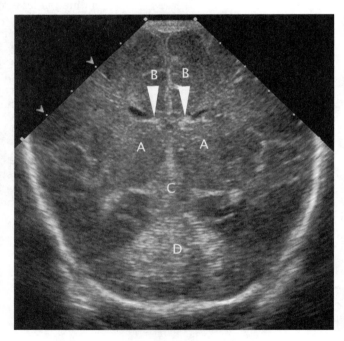

2. Coronal brain

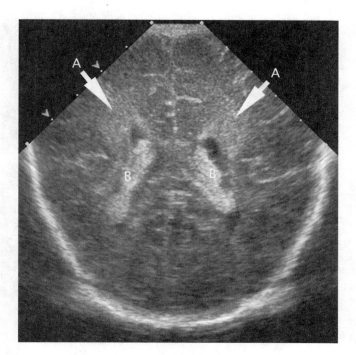

3. Coronal brain

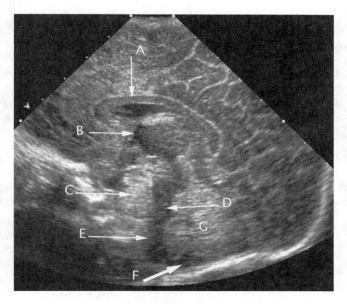

4. Sagittal midline brain

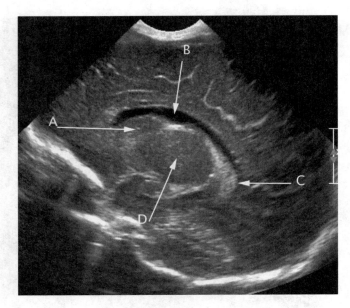

5. Parasagittal brain

CHAPTER REVIEW

Multiple Choice

Complete each question by circling the best answer.

1. Which of the following is the primary acoustic window used to image the neonatal brain?
   a. mastoid fontanelle
   b. anterior fontanelle
   c. posterior fontanelle
   d. superficial fontanelle

2. Excessive pressure on the anterior fontanelle during the examination may cause what?
   a. tachycardia
   b. respiratory arrest
   c. bradycardia
   d. image artifacts

3. Which of the following is NOT one of the meninges that cover and protect the brain and spinal cord?
   a. pia mater
   b. dura mater
   c. arachnoid
   d. vergae mater

4. Which of the following is NOT one of the four cortical lobes of the brain?
   a. frontal
   b. thalamus
   c. parietal
   d. temporal

5. Which of the following is NOT contained in the posterior fossa?
   a. third ventricle
   b. fourth ventricle
   c. cerebellum
   d. brainstem

6. Which of the following statements regarding the neonatal brain is FALSE?
   a. Coronal scanning allows for a comparison of the echogenicity between the choroid plexus and the periventricular parenchyma.
   b. The echogenicity of the periventricular white matter should be slightly brighter than the choroid plexus.
   c. Changes in echogenicity in this area should arouse suspicion for hemorrhage or infarct.
   d. Evaluating this area through the posterior fontanelle may also be helpful.

7. Which of the following statements regarding the premature brain is FALSE?
   a. In very premature infants, the cavum vergae is often seen.
   b. In premature infants, the cisterna magna should still be seen.
   c. Widely spaced sylvian fissures on the coronal view is a marker of extreme prematurity.
   d. The sulci are easily visible, even in a very premature infant.

8. A sonogram of the neonatal brain in a preterm infant demonstrates a thickened and irregular left choroid plexus. Echogenic material is also noted in the left occipital horn of the lateral ventricle. What grade of GM-IVH would be assigned to this patient?

   a. grade I
   b. grade II
   c. grade III
   d. grade IV

9. The sonogram on the neonatal brain of a preterm infant demonstrates a focal hyperechoic area anterior to the caudothalamic groove on the parasagittal view bilaterally. The ventricles are not dilated and no other abnormalities are seen. What grade of GM-IVH would be assigned to this patient?

   a. grade I
   b. grade II
   c. grade III
   d. grade IV

10. A sonogram is performed on a premature infant 2 days after delivery. An echogenic area is seen in the frontal lobe of the brain. On a follow-up examination, a cystic space is noted in the same area. What grade of GM-IVH would be assigned to this patient?

    a. grade I
    b. grade II
    c. grade III
    d. grade IV

11. Which of the following statements regarding Grade I GM-IVH is FALSE?

    a. The hemorrhage may be unilateral or bilateral.
    b. Ventricular dilatation does not occur with Grade I GM-IVH.
    c. Patients with Grade I GM-IVH will experience developmental delays and seizures.
    d. Over time the clot will evolve and demonstrate a cystic center.

12. Which of the following statements regarding grade II GM-IVH is FALSE?

    a. The ventricles are dilated in Grade II GM-IVH.
    b. Grade II GM-IVH occurs when hemorrhage ruptures through the ependymal lining and enters the ventricular cavity.
    c. Blood typically accumulates and migrates to the most dependent occipital horn.
    d. Scanning through the posterior fontanelle can aid in visualizing the occipital horn.

13. A sonogram of the neonatal head in a preterm infant demonstrates echogenic material filling a dilated right lateral ventricle. The lining of the ventricle is thickened and echogenic as well. What grade of GM-IVH would be assigned to this patient?

    a. grade I
    b. grade II
    c. grade III
    d. grade IV

14. A fluid-filled space that has replaced normal brain parenchyma due to the result of a destructive process such as an intraparenchymal hemorrhage is called what?

    a. anencephaly
    b. meningocele
    c. porencephaly
    d. myelomeningocele

15. A 4-week old premature infant presents for a sonogram of the brain. Small, cystic structures are visualized in the periventricular area of the brain bilaterally. What is the most likely cause of this finding?

    a. hydrocephalus
    b. grade III GM-IVH
    c. cerebellar hemorrhage
    d. periventricular leukomalacia

16. A dilatation of the ventricular system that results from impairment of cerebral spinal fluid dynamics or brain parenchymal loss is called:

    a. anencephaly.
    b. holoprosencephaly.
    c. porencephaly.
    d. hydrocephalus.

17. Which of the following acoustic windows provides the best approach for visualizing cerebellar hemorrhage?

    a. mastoid fontanelle
    b. anterior fontanelle
    c. posterior fontanelle
    d. superficial fontanelle

18. Which term describes the softening of white matter of the brain that occurs with ischemia?

    a. holoprosencephaly
    b. leukomalacia
    c. hydrocephalus
    d. intraventricular hemorrhage

19. A sonogram of the neonatal brain demonstrates widely separated frontal horns of the lateral ventricles. The third ventricle is displaced upward between the frontal horns. On a midline sagittal image, the medial sulci and gyri are arranged radially in the classic "sunburst sign." What pathology will cause these findings?
    a. holoprosencephaly
    b. Dandy–Walker complex
    c. absence of the corpus callosum
    d. hydrocephalus

20. Which of the following is the most severe form of holoprosencephaly?
    a. alobar holoprosencephaly
    b. lobar holoprosencephaly
    c. semilobar holoprosencephaly
    d. all forms have the same severity

Fill-in-the-Blank

1. Closure of the anterior fontanelle begins at about _____ of age and is usually complete by _____ of age.

2. Two alternative acoustic windows are the _____ fontanelle and the _____ fontanelle. When evaluating the neonatal brain, images are obtained in the _____ and _____ planes.

3. The central nervous system is made up of the _____ and _____ _____. _____ fluid surrounds and protects the CNS.

4. Three protective membranes called _____ cover and protect the brain and spinal cord. The _____ is the outer layer that attaches to the inside of the cranial vault. The _____ surrounds the surface of the cerebral cortex and the _____ is interposed between the two.

5. The brain is divided into the _____, _____, and _____.

6. The ventricular system is comprised of the paired _____ ventricles and the midline _____ and _____ ventricles.

7. When evaluating the brain via the anterior fontanelle in the coronal plane, images are obtained by angling the transducer from the _____ lobe to the posterior _____ cortex. The _____ of the brain is projected on the left side of the image.

8. In the sagittal plane, the transducer is angled _____ to _____ through each cerebral hemisphere. By convention, the _____ aspect of the brain is placed on the left side of the image.

9. Nearly all premature infants show an increased _____ in the parenchymal region around the peritrigonal area of the ventricles. This is termed the _____ _____ _____ _____. Scanning through the _____ fontanelle places the fiber tracts more parallel to the beam and can aid in the diagnosis.

10. The majority of germinal matrix intraventricular hemorrhages occur within the _____ of life. Preterm neonates with a birth weight less than _____ and a gestational age of less than _____ have the greatest risk for developing cerebral events such as ICH.

11. Intracranial hemorrhage is divided into _____ grades. The area of the _____ groove is the primary site for hemorrhage in the preterm infant.

12. Grade III GM-IVH consists of _____ with _____. The lining of the ventricles may become _____ and _____ due to irritation from the breakdown of blood products. Posthemorrhagic _____ is often a complication.

13. If an obstruction occurs within the ventricular system, it is referred to as _____ hydrocephalus, whereas if it occurs outside the ventricular system, the term _____ hydrocephalus is used.

14. When scanning through the mastoid fontanelle in the coronal plane, the transducer notch is pointed toward the _____ _____. For an axial view, the transducer is positioned with the notch toward the _____ _____.

15. _____ _____ is the most common hypoxic-ischemic brain injury in the premature infant. It appears as an increased _____ and is almost always _____ and _____.

16. When evaluating for subdural or subarachnoid fluid collections, a high-frequency _____ array transducer should be used. Fluid in the subarachnoid space displaces cortical vessels away from the _____ _____ toward the _____ _____, whereas fluid in the subdural space displaces cortical vessels toward the _____ _____ and contains no _____ _____.

17. Dandy–Walker malformation is characterized by cystic dilatation of the _____ _____, superior elevation of the _____, partial or complete absence of the _____, and small _____ hemispheres.

18. Type _____ Chiari malformation is the most common type seen in infants and neonates and is nearly always associated with _____. It is associated with a small _____ _____, downward displacement of the _____, _____, and _____ _____ into the upper spinal canal.

19. The most common intracranial vascular anomaly presenting in the neonatal period is the _____ _____ _____. Sonographically, this presents as a well-circumscribed, anechoic mass in the _____ posterior to the _____ _____. Color Doppler demonstrates _____ flow within the malformation.

20. Holoprosencephaly occurs when the primitive forebrain fails to divide into two separate _____ _____. Midline _____ anomalies are also associated with these malformations.

Short Answer

1. When performing an examination on a preterm infant, what precautions are taken to limit the risk of infection and stress to the infant?

2. When evaluating the brain in a very premature infant, what sonographic features of prematurity should be understood to avoid misdiagnosis of pathology?

3. Why is intracranial hemorrhage common in premature infants but low in infants born after the 36th week of gestation?

4. List the clinical signs of hydrocephalus.

5. Describe the technique used to evaluate infants with suspected elevated intracranial pressure using spectral Doppler.

IMAGE EVALUATION/PATHOLOGY

Review the images and answer the following questions.

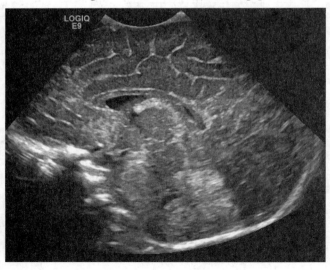

1. Was this sagittal image of the brain taken in a term or premature infant? How can you tell?

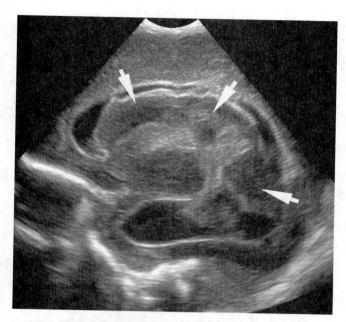

2. What are the *arrows* pointing to in this sagittal image of the brain in a premature infant? How would you classify this and why?

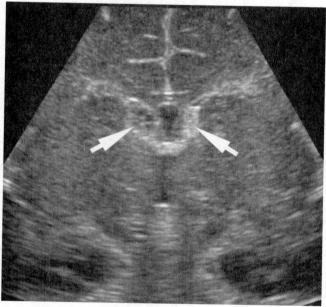

3. What are the *arrows* pointing to in this coronal image of the brain in a premature infant? How would you classify this and why?

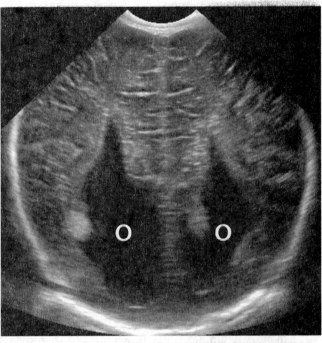

4. A prenatal sonogram showed abnormalities in the fetal brain. After delivery, a sonogram of the brain was ordered. The third ventricle was displaced upward and the frontal horns of the lateral ventricles were noted to be separated widely. What is seen in this coronal image? Given these findings, what is the most likely diagnosis?

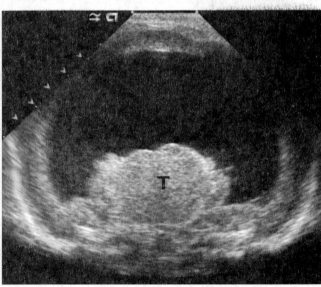

5. This infant was born with severe midline facial anomalies. A sonogram of the neonatal brain was ordered. What is seen in this coronal image? What is the likely diagnosis?

CASE STUDIES

Review the images and answer the following questions.

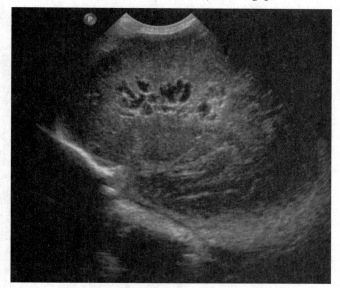

1. An infant presented for a sonogram of the brain following a traumatic delivery. During the sonogram, echogenic areas were noted bilaterally in the periventricular parenchyma. A follow-up sonogram was performed one month after delivery. This sagittal image was taken lateral to the right lateral ventricle. What is seen in this image? What is the likely diagnosis?

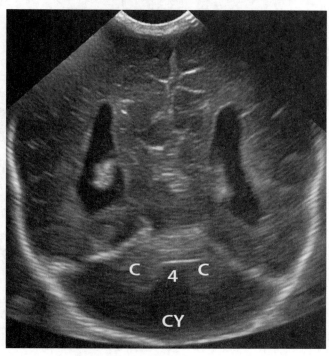

2. A neonate presents after delivery for a sonogram of the brain following an abnormal prenatal sonogram. Describe what is seen in this coronal image of the brain. What is the most likely diagnosis

The Infant Spine

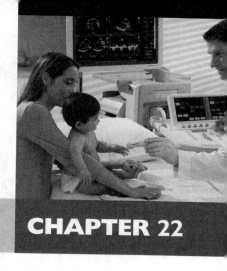

REVIEW OF GLOSSARY TERMS

Matching

Match the terms with their definitions.

KEY TERMS

1. _____ cauda equina

2. _____ conus medullaris

3. _____ dura

4. _____ dysraphism

5. _____ epidural space

6. _____ filum terminale

7. _____ hydromelia

8. _____ myelomalacia

9. _____ syrinx

DEFINITION

a. Tapering end of the spinal cord, caudal to the conus medullaris
b. Outermost layer of the covering of the spinal cord
c. Collection of nerve roots at the end of the spinal column; includes lumbar and sacral nerve roots
d. Anomalies associated with incomplete fusion of the neural tube during embryological development
e. Fluid-filled cavity in the spinal cord
f. Space between the outermost layer of the spinal cord, the dura, and the spinal column
g. The most caudal portion of the spinal cord
h. Softening of the spinal cord frequently caused by a lack of blood supply
i. Dilatation of the central canal of the spinal cord

ANATOMY AND PHYSIOLOGY REVIEW

Image Labeling

Complete the labels in the images that follow.

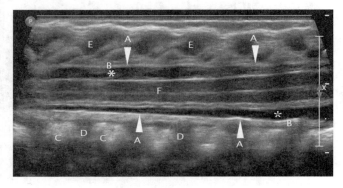

1. Sagittal spine

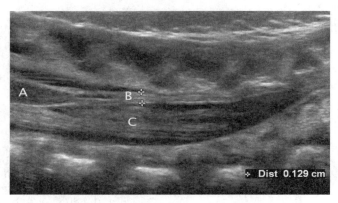

2. Sagittal spine

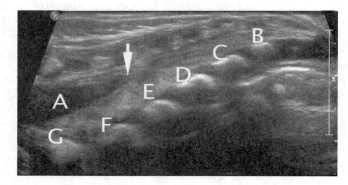

3. Sagittal spine

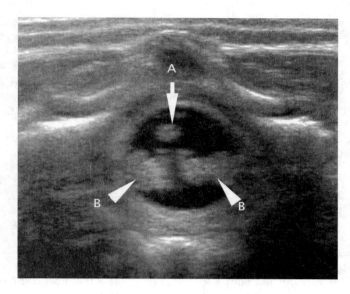

4. Transverse spine

CHAPTER REVIEW

Multiple Choice

Complete each question by circling the best answer.

1. Sonography of the spine is limited to infants under what age?
   a. 1 month
   b. 2 months
   c. 6 months
   d. 12 months

2. At which level does the normal spinal cord taper to a point and terminate with the conus medularis?
   a. S1–L5
   b. L4–L5
   c. L3–L4
   d. L1–L2

3. Which of the following statements regarding the sonographic anatomy of the spinal cord is FALSE?
   a. In the axial plane, the filum terminale appears as a round, echogenic nerve arising from the tip of the conus.
   b. The nerves of the cauda equina appear as smaller, echogenic dots surrounding the conus and filum.
   c. The cord is surrounded by CSF, which is contained by the echogenic dura surrounding the canal.
   d. The spinal cord is seen as a hyperechoic structure located within the spinal canal.

4. How many vertebrae make up the sacral spine?
   a. one
   b. three
   c. five
   d. seven

5. How many vertebrae make up the lumbar spine?
   a. one
   b. three
   c. five
   d. seven

6. How many vertebrae make up the thoracic spine?
   a. five
   b. eight
   c. ten
   d. twelve

7. While performing an evaluation of the spine on an infant, a small, cystic structure is seen inferior to the tip of the conus medularis. No other defect is seen. What is the most likely cause of this structure?
   a. filar cyst
   b. tethered cord
   c. meningocele
   d. diastomyelia

8. What is the most common location for a spinal dysraphism?
   a. cervical spine
   b. thoracic spine
   c. lumbosacral spine
   d. dysraphisms occur equally throughout the spine

9. Which of the following closed spinal dysraphisms does NOT present as a subcutaneous mass?
   a. lipomyelocele
   b. tethered cord
   c. lipomyelomeningocele
   d. myelocystocele

10. What is the defect that occurs when there is a failure of the spinal cord to fold into a neural tube, and presents with the skin, musculature, and bony vertebral arches splayed laterally to the defect?
    a. terminal myelocystocele
    b. myelomeningocele
    c. dorsal dermal sinus
    d. diastomyelia

11. Which of the following is a condition in which the spinal cord is separated into two hemicords?
    a. terminal myelocystocele
    b. myelomeningocele
    c. dorsal dermal sinus
    d. diastomyelia

12. Which of the following statements regarding tethered cord are FALSE?
    a. A tethered cord is associated with dysraphic spinal anomalies.
    b. A tethered cord is low-lying with a thickened filum terminale.
    c. Symptoms may not present until the child grows and the cord is pulled tight.
    d. The cord and nerve roots will have increased motion.

13. The conus is considered abnormally low at or below which level?
    a. L1
    b. L2
    c. L3
    d. L5

14. In which region of the spine does diastomyelia most commonly occur?
    a. cervical
    b. cervicothoracic
    c. thoracolumbar
    d. lumbosacral

15. Which of the following is a condition that represents a very focal disruption in the development or fusion of the spinal canal and presents with a thin tract that travels from the skin to the spinal canal?
    a. terminal myelocystocele
    b. myelomeningocele
    c. dorsal dermal sinus
    d. diastomyelia

16. Which condition are patients with a dorsal dermal sinus at risk of developing?
    a. meningitis
    b. spinal lipoma
    c. paralysis
    d. scoliosis

17. What is the most common indication for a spinal sonogram?
    a. palpable mass
    b. sacral dimple or pit
    c. visible defect
    d. neurological deficits

18. An infant presents for a spinal sonogram with a palpable, skin-covered mass in the lumbar region. During the evaluation, a bony defect is seen and an echogenic fatty mass is seen to be contained within the spinal canal. The mass appears to distort and tether the spinal cord. What is the most likely diagnosis?
    a. intradural lipoma
    b. lipoma of the filum terminale
    c. lipomyelomeningocele
    d. lipomyelocele

19. Which of the following is a dilated central canal?
    a. hydromelia
    b. myelocystocele
    c. diastomyelia
    d. myelomeningocele

20. A patient presents for a spinal sonogram with a sacral dimple. A hypoechoic tract is visualized extending from the skin to a cystic structure. Neither the hypoechoic tract nor the cystic collection appears to be connected to the spine. No other abnormalities are seen. What is the most likely diagnosis?
    a. myelocystocele
    b. pilonidal cyst
    c. myelomeningocele
    d. diastomyelia

Fill-in-the-Blank

1. The value of sonography of the spine decreases at _____ and is nearly nondiagnostic after _____, due to ossification of the _____ spinous processes.

2. The infant spine is examined from the _____ junction to the _____. The level of the _____ _____, as well as the position of the _____ _____ in the spinal canal, is documented.

3. During the examination, _____ and _____ _____ motion should be detected and noted.

4. Sonographically, the spinal cord is _____, whereas the arachnoid-dural layer is _____ _____ and is seen lining the canal both anteriorly and posteriorly. The cerebrospinal fluid is _____ and is seen surrounding the cord.

5. The spine is larger in the _____ and _____ regions, due to the amount of _____ in these areas.

6. The conus gives way to the _____ _____, which is surrounded by the echogenic strands of the _____ _____.

7. Spinal _____ refers to a spinal abnormality caused by inadequate or improper fusion of the neural tube early in life. They are characterized as _____ if neural tissue is exposed without covering or _____ if the defect is covered by skin.

8. A _____ presents as a flat plate of neural tissue flush with the skin surface, whereas in the _____, the neural plate is elevated above the skin surface, due to an enlarged, underlying subarachnoid space.

9. A tethered cord is a low-lying cord with a thickened _____ _____. This can cause decreased _____ _____, _____, and _____ function.

10. Patients with _____ or _____ malformations or _____ syndrome have a high association with tethered cord.

11. The conus is considered abnormally low at or below the level of _____. The cord and nerve roots will have _____ motion. The _____ _____ may also be abnormally thick.

12. _____ is the separation of the spinal cord into two hemicords separated by a _____ or _____ septum. It is associated with _____ cord, _____, _____, _____ anomalies, and dilatation of the central canal.

13. A dorsal dermal sinus manifests clinically as a deep _____ _____ that should not be confused with a _____ _____ located in the gluteal fold.

14. Spinal lipomas include _____, _____, _____ _____, and lipomas of the _____ _____.

15. Sonography of the spine may be done to evaluate for birth trauma especially following a difficult _____

    delivery. Cord injury may manifest sonographically as cord _____, _____, and

    _____ outside the cord.

Short Answer

1. Describe the appropriate transducer selection and patient positioning used for sonographic evaluation of the neonatal spine.

2. List the closed dysraphisms that can present with a cutaneous marker. What types of cutaneous markers are associated with spinal dysraphisms?

3. Describe the most common method of determining the level of the conus medullaris and exact localization of any intraspinal abnormalities.

IMAGE EVALUATION/PATHOLOGY

Review the images and answer the following questions.

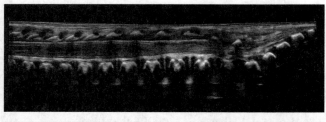

1. Where does the conus end in this sagittal panoramic image of the neonatal spine?

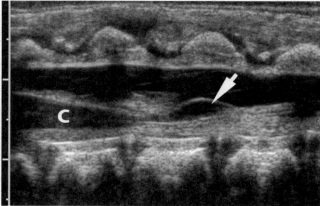

2. What is the *arrow* pointing to in this image? Where is this structure located?

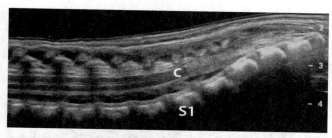

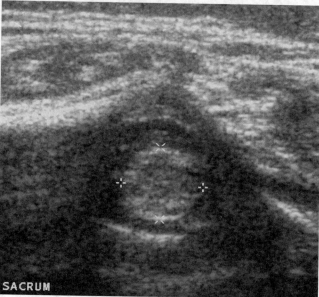

3. Where does the conus end in this sagittal panoramic image of the neonatal spine? What is this condition called? When is the conus considered abnormally low?

4. Describe what is seen in this transverse image taken at the level of the sacrum. What is the likely diagnosis?

CASE STUDY

Review the images and answer the following questions.

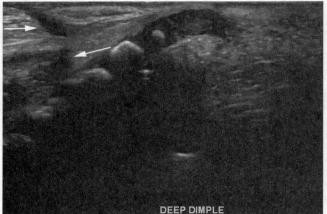

DEEP DIMPLE

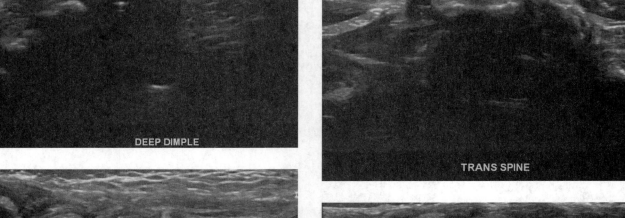

TRANS SPINE

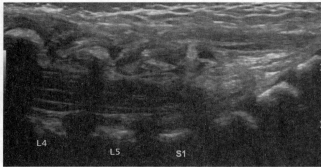

L4   L5   S1

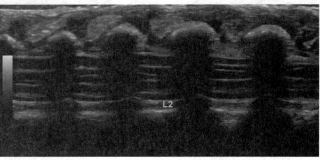

L2

1. An infant presents for a sonogram of the spine with the clinical finding of a deep midline dimple. Describe what is seen in the images. Is the spinal cord tethered?

The Infant Hip Joint

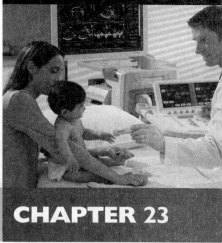

REVIEW OF GLOSSARY TERMS

Matching

Match the terms with their definitions.

KEY TERMS

1. _____ abduct

2. _____ adduct

3. _____ arthrocentesis

4. _____ erythrocyte sedimentation rate

5. _____ mesoderm

6. _____ oligohydramnios

7. _____ osteomyelitis

8. _____ torticollis

DEFINITION

a. Infection of the bone marrow and bone
b. To move away from the midline
c. The middle germ cell layer that contributes to the embryologic development of connective tissue, bone, blood, muscle, vessels, and lymphatics
d. To move toward the midline
e. A head that is held sideways due to muscle contraction
f. To remove fluid from a joint through a needle
g. A decreased amount of amniotic fluid around the fetus
h. Laboratory test that is a nonspecific indicator for inflammation

ANATOMY AND PHYSIOLOGY REVIEW

Image Labeling

Complete the labels in the images that follow.

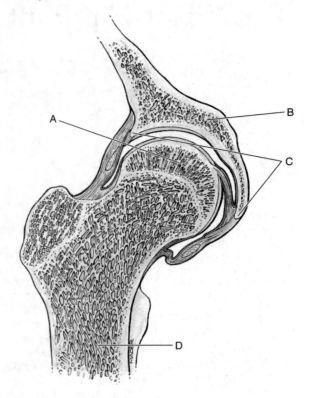

1. Anterior hip joint

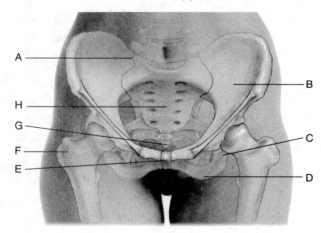

2. Female bony pelvis

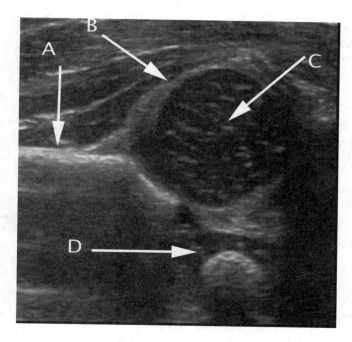

3. Sonographic anatomy

CHAPTER REVIEW

Multiple Choice

Complete each question by circling the best answer.

1. What are the two most common methods used to evaluate for DDH?
   a. clinical assessment and MRI
   b. clinical assessment and sonography
   c. sonography and X-ray
   d. sonography and laparoscopic evaluation

2. Which germ cell layer are the bones, connective tissues, and muscles derived from?
   a. ectoderm
   b. endoderm
   c. mesoderm
   d. zygoderm

3. When does DDH occur most commonly?
   a. at birth
   b. at 2 months of age
   c. at 4 months of age
   d. at 8 months of age

4. Which of the following is NOT a risk factor for developing DDH?
   a. babies born in the breech position
   b. positive family history
   c. high birth weight
   d. polyhydramnios

5. In which of the following maneuvers does the examiner attempt to push the femoral head out of the socket?
   a. Ortolani maneuver
   b. Barlow maneuver
   c. Murphy maneuver
   d. Whitlow maneuver

6. Which of the following statements regarding the alpha angle is FALSE?
   a. The alpha angle is defined as the bony roof of the acetabulum.
   b. The alpha angle is obtained in the transverse plane.
   c. The alpha angle is the primary measure of hip dysplasia.
   d. When the alpha angle is greater than 60 degrees, it is considered normal.

7. Which of the following statements regarding evaluation of the hips is FALSE?
   a. The coronal plane can be used to assess how well the femoral head is contained within the acetabulum.
   b. A dislocated hip will sit completely out of the acetabulum.
   c. The lower limit for normal femoral head coverage is 45%.
   d. Assessing femoral head coverage is the most reproducible method for diagnosing DDH.

8. Which condition is described if a hip demonstrates posterior, superior, and lateral displacement of the femoral head during flexion?
   a. dislocated
   b. subluxed
   c. normal
   d. inflamed

9. Which of the following statements regarding the transverse scan plane is FALSE?
   a. The transverse scan plan may be obtained in a neutral or flexed position.
   b. The alpha and beta angles are taken in this plane.
   c. Stress maneuvers are performed in the transverse plane.
   d. If the hip is dislocated, the normal U configuration will not be identified.

10. A 3-year-old patient presents with a low-grade fever and refusal to bear weight on her left hip. She recently had an upper respiratory infection. What is the MOST likely diagnosis?
    a. septic arthritis
    b. hip dislocation
    c. DDH
    d. transient synovitis

Fill-in-the-Blank

1. Developmental dysplasia of the hip describes a range of dysplasia including: _____, _____, and frank _____.

2. The frequency of DDH is _____ in _____.

3. The hip bone is composed of the _____, _____, and _____.

4. The rounded femoral head sits in the _____.

5. The femoral head is composed of _____ at birth. It begins to ossify from the center outward between _____ months.

6. During fetal development, _____ _____ contribute to the laxity of fetal ligaments.

7. An _____ _____ is considered a strong positive Barlow and Ortolani sign.

8. Imaging is performed with and without _____. Imaging planes include the _____ plane without _____ and the _____ plane with and without _____.

9. In the coronal scan plan, the femoral head is seen sitting in the _____. The _____ _____ should appear as a straight line.

10. An alpha angle of greater than or equal to _____ is considered normal.

11. In a coronal/flexion image of the hip, the hip has a ball-on-a-spoon appearance. The ball is the _____ _____, the _____ _____ represents the handle of the spoon, and the scoop of the spoon is the _____.

12. In the transverse scan plan, the _____ _____ and the _____ form a U or V configuration around the _____ _____.

13. When a child presents with hip pain, fever, limited movement, and refusal to bear weight, sonography can be used to evaluate for the presence of a _____ _____.

14. _____ _____ can be treated with anti-inflammatory medication and rest, whereas _____ _____ is a more serious bacterial infection that is typically treated with intravenous antibiotics.

15. When evaluating for a hip effusion, the normal hip capsule has a _____ appearance, whereas if an effusion is present the capsule bulges _____. An abnormal appearance is defined as a capsular thickness greater than _____ mm.

Short Answer

1. How does the composition of the femoral head affect the ability to perform a diagnostic sonogram of the infant hip?

2. What risk factors are associated with DDH?

3. What physical characteristics may indicate an infant has DDH?

4. Why is sonography of the infant's hips typically performed at 4 to 6 weeks of age and not earlier?

IMAGE EVALUATION/PATHOLOGY

Review the images and answer the following questions.

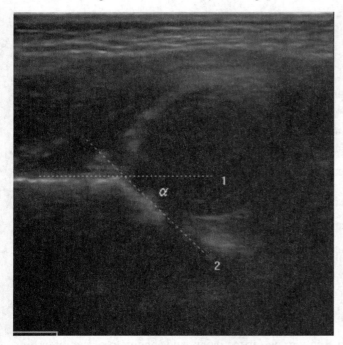

1. This 3-month-old patient presents with an abnormal physical examination. What is being measured in this image? What is the purpose of this measurement?

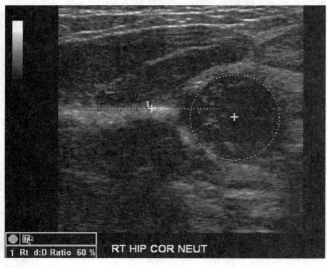

2. What is being measured in this image? Is this measurement considered normal?

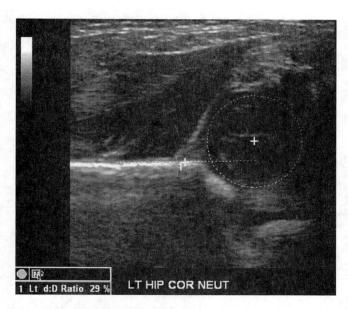

LT HIP COR NEUT
1 Lt d:D Ratio 29 %

3. What is being measured in this image? Is this measurement considered normal?

4. A 3-year-old patient presents with fever and pain in the left hip. What is seen in this image of the hip?

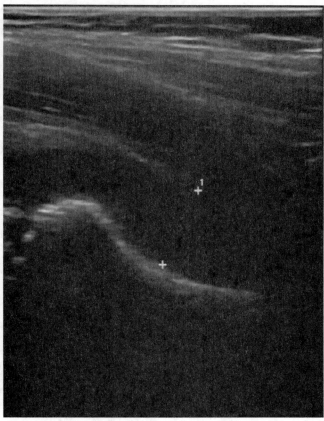

CASE STUDY

Review the image and answer the following question.

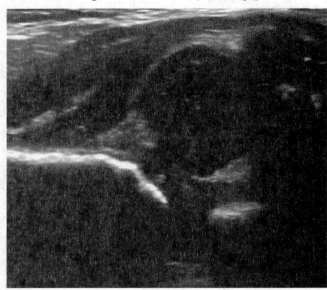

1. A 10-week-old girl presents with an abnormal physical examination for a sonogram of the hips. Describe what is seen in this image.

PART 4

SPECIAL STUDY SONOGRAPHY

Organ Transplantation

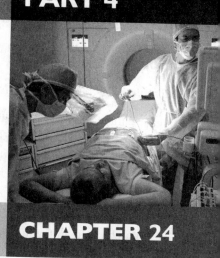

REVIEW OF GLOSSARY TERMS

Matching

Match the terms with their definitions.

KEY TERMS

1. _____ allograft

2. _____ heterotopically

3. _____ histocompatibility

4. _____ immunosuppressive medication

DEFINITION

a. Pharmaceutical agents prescribed to prevent or decrease the immune response
b. Graft transplanted between genetically nonidentical individuals of the same species
c. Occurring in an abnormal place
d. State of a donor and recipient sharing a sufficient number of histocompatibility antigens so an allograft is accepted and remains functional

ANATOMY AND PHYSIOLOGY REVIEW

Image Labeling

Complete the labels in the images that follow.

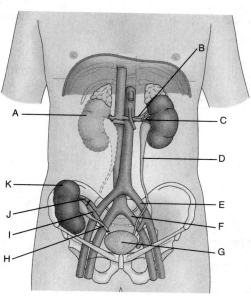

1. Anatomy of kidney transplant

CHAPTER REVIEW

Multiple Choice

Complete each question by circling the best answer.

1. A patient who has uremia may be a candidate for which type of organ transplant?
   a. liver
   b. kidney
   c. pancreas
   d. lung

2. Which of the following is NOT a common cause of liver transplant?
   a. diabetes
   b. hepatitis C
   c. cirrhosis
   d. alcoholic liver disease

3. Which of the following is NOT a contraindication to liver transplantation?
   a. sepsis
   b. metastatic cancer
   c. active substance abuse
   d. all of the above are contraindications to liver transplantation

4. A patient with which of the following conditions is MOST likely to be a candidate for pancreas transplant?
   a. alcoholism
   b. uremia
   c. uncontrolled diabetes
   d. cystic fibrosis

5. Which of the following laboratory values are used to evaluate the function of a renal allograft?
   a. AST and ALT
   b. PT and INR
   c. amylase and lipase
   d. BUN and creatinine

6. Which of the following is NOT a fluid collection that can cause compression of the vascular flow to a renal allograft?
   a. biloma
   b. hematoma
   c. lymphocele
   d. urinoma

7. Which of the following is a condition that affects renal function and is more common in cadaveric grafts?
   a. acute accelerated rejection
   b. acute tubular necrosis
   c. lymphocele
   d. polymona-BK virus nephropathy

8. Which of the following is typically seen as a result of biopsy trauma in a renal allograft?
   a. lymphocele
   b. abscess
   c. arteriovenous malformation
   d. urinoma

9. What is the most significant liver allograft pathology?
   a. biliary sludge
   b. biloma
   c. hepatic artery stenosis
   d. biliary strictures

10. What is the gold standard for evaluation of renal allograft rejection?
    a. sonography
    b. core biopsy
    c. computed tomography
    d. nuclear medicine

Fill-in-the-Blank

1. Following an organ transplant, patients are typically on two types of medication: _____ and _____. Levels that are too low can lead to _____, whereas higher levels can cause _____.

2. The one-year survival rate for a liver transplant is _____ %, a simultaneous pancreas and kidney transplant is _____ % successful, a pancreas transplant following a renal transplant is _____ % successful, and a pancreas transplant alone is only _____ % effective.

3. There are two types of organ donations, either a _____ donor or one harvested from a _____.

4. A pancreatic allograft is placed either in the _____, where it is oriented _____ _____, or _____ abdomen, where it is oriented _____.

5. The surgery for a liver allograft requires _____ vascular connections, as well as a _____ anastomosis.

6. A liver allograft from a live donor involves a right hepatectomy of segments _____, along with the right _____ vein.

7. A renal allograft has an average life span of _____ years; however, a living donor organ has a life span of _____ years.

8. A renal allograft must be evaluated sonographically for its _____ and overall _____, as well as thickness of the _____.

9. Chronic rejection of a renal allograft occurs after _____ months. The kidney begins to _____ and interstitial _____ becomes noticeable sonographically.

10. Spectral Doppler tracings of the _____ arteries should be obtained from the upper, mid, and lower poles of the renal allograft. An RI ≤ _____ and or a pulsatility index ≤ _____ are considered normal.

11. Two sonographic signs of rejection of a pancreatic allograft include a _____ echotexture and an overall _____ in graft size.

12. Fluid collections surrounding a liver allograft should resolve within _____ days postoperatively.

13. Renal artery _____ leads to diminished flow to the renal allograft and causes a _____ in the size of the allograft. Spectral Doppler will demonstrate a peak systolic velocity > _____ c/s with distant _____.

14. Biliary strictures in a liver allograft present clinically with _____ _____ and abnormal _____ _____ _____. Biliary stasis can lead to ascending _____.

15. Hepatic _____ thrombosis and stenosis are major clinical concerns in liver allografts. Evaluation of the portal vein must demonstrate _____ flow.

Short Answer

1. Describe the typical location for the placement of a renal allograft. What is a heterotopic renal transplant?

2. Describe the changes that can be seen sonographically in a renal allograft when acute accelerated rejection or acute tubular necrosis is present.

3. Why is it important to cross-match and type the HLA of the donor and recipient prior to organ transplantation?

IMAGE EVALUATION/PATHOLOGY

Review the images and answer the following questions.

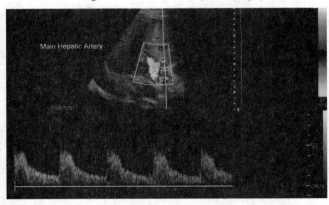

1. What vessel is being interrogated in this image? Does the waveform appear normal? Why is it important to evaluate flow in this vessel?

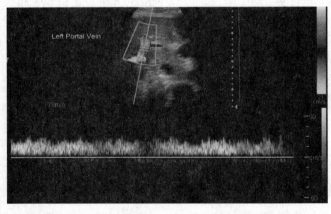

2. What vessel is being interrogated in this image? Does this waveform appear normal? What direction of flow is normal in this vessel?

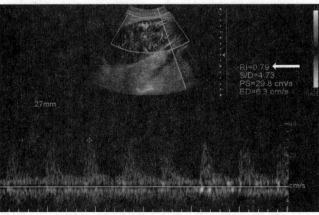

3. What measurements are recorded in this image? What is the normal value for the RI in a renal allograft?

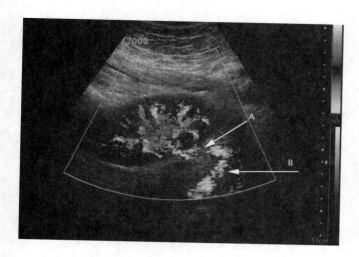

4. What vessels are the arrows (*A*) and (*B*) pointing to in this image of a renal allograft?

Point-of-Care Sonography

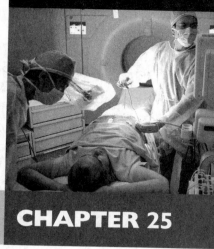

REVIEW OF GLOSSARY TERMS

Matching

Match the terms with their definitions.

KEY TERMS

1. _____ cardiac tamponade

2. _____ deep vein thrombosis

3. _____ diagnostic peritoneal lavage

4. _____ hemoperitoneum

5. _____ hemothorax

6. _____ laparotomy

7. _____ parietal pleura

8. _____ pericardial effusion

9. _____ pleural effusion

DEFINITION

a. Pleura that lines the inner chest walls and covers the diaphragm

b. The presence of extravasated blood in the peritoneal cavity

c. Mechanical compression of the heart resulting from large amounts of fluid collecting in the pericardial space, limiting the heart's normal range of motion

d. Presence of fluid in the pleural cavity

e. A procedure in which an incision is made in the abdomen to insert a camera to visualize the abdomen and pelvic structures and spaces

f. Presence of fluid within the pericardium

g. Surgical procedure used to insert a catheter through the abdominal wall and fascia; used to evaluate for bleeding in the abdomen

h. The formation or presence of a thrombus within a vein

i. Accumulation of blood in the pleural cavity

ANATOMY AND PHYSIOLOGY REVIEW

Image Labeling

Complete the labels in the images that follow.

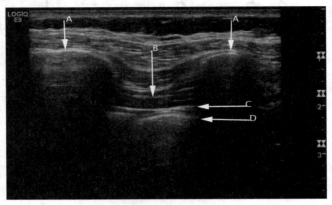

1. Anatomy of the thorax

CHAPTER REVIEW

Multiple Choice

Complete each question by circling the best answer.

1. What is the main purpose of the FAST exam?
   a. Evaluate for gallstones and kidney stones.
   b. Perform a complete abdominal sonogram in as little time as possible.
   c. Evaluate for free fluid or blood in the abdomen following trauma.
   d. Evaluate for life-threatening conditions such as AAA and appendicitis.

2. The primary purpose of the eFAST is to extend the search to determine what sequelae of trauma?
   a. pleural effusion
   b. pericardial effusion
   c. cardiac tamponade
   d. pneumothorax

3. Which of the following is NOT evaluated in cases of the emergency cardiac examination?
   a. pericardial fluid
   b. diagnosis of mitral valve prolapse
   c. detection of cardiac motion in patients with pulseless electrical activity
   d. evaluation of tamponade

4. Which of the following is NOT one of the most common acoustic windows used in emergency echocardiography?
   a. suprasternal
   b. parasternal
   c. apical
   d. subxiphoid

5. What is fluid surrounding the heart and located within the pericardial sac called?
   a. ascites
   b. pleural effusion
   c. pericardial effusion
   d. pneumothorax

6. Which of the following statements regarding pericardial effusion is FALSE?
   a. Blood can collect between the visceral and parietal layers.
   b. Rapid hemorrhage can cause hypertension.
   c. A decrease in right heart filling can be noted.
   d. Decreased left ventricular stroke volume is possible.

7. A 32-year-old patient presents to the emergency room following a serious motor vehicle accident. What condition is demonstrated if fluid is noted around the heart and the intraventricular septum appears to bow into the left ventricle?

   a. pleural effusion
   b. pneumothorax
   c. cardiac tamponade
   d. pulseless cardiac activity

8. Which of the following is the most sensitive at detecting pneumothorax?

   a. sonography
   b. physical examination
   c. patient complaints
   d. chest radiography

9. A patient presents to the emergency room with a history of trauma to the chest. When evaluating the thorax, you visualize the "gliding sign" as the patient breathes in and out. This sign is appreciated bilaterally. What does this represent?

   a. This sign is not used to evaluate for chest pathology.
   b. This sign is normal; no pneumothorax is seen.
   c. This patient has bilateral pneumothorax and requires immediate intervention.
   d. The represents a cardiac tamponade and requires immediate intervention.

10. A patient with a pneumothorax will present with absent lung sliding on real-time sonography. Which of the following conditions CANNOT cause this finding?

   a. acute respiratory distress syndrome
   b. mainstem intubation
   c. pleural embolism
   d. pleural adhesions

Fill-in-the-Blank

1. Many life-threatening injuries cause bleeding in the _____, _____, _____, and _____ regions.

2. The primary purpose of the FAST exam is a methodical search for free _____ or _____ in the dependent portions of the _____, _____ spaces, _____ spaces, and the _____.

3. With the transducer oriented transversely in the subxiphoid region, the _____ _____ image can be seen. The _____ of the heart including both atria should be located on the patient's right side. The _____ of the heart is located more to the patient's left side.

4. Two layers of pericardium surround the heart, the _____ pericardium and the _____ pericardium. Up to _____ mL of normal serous fluid can collect within the pericardial sac.

5. In the subxiphoid window, blood will most often be noted _____ or posteriorly as it outlines the free wall of the left atria and ventricle.

6. With cardiac tamponade the outer wall of the ventricles depress _____. The intraventricular septum bows into the _____ ventricle, which is known as _____ _____ _____.

7. In normal patients, a sliding motion can be seen and is caused by the movement of the _____ pleura during respiration along the static _____ pleura. This is seen as an _____ line that moves with respiration.

8. The normal, back-and-forth movement of the pleural layers causes a _____ sign or a _____ sign. Absence of sliding indicates there is a _____. The more _____ location is the common site for pneumothorax.

9. On M-mode, the normal sliding lung will demonstrate a _____ sign. In the case of pneumothorax, the M-mode will reveal a series of _____ _____ lines called the _____ or _____ sign.

10. The phenomenon of demonstrating absent lung sliding and normal lung sliding occurring between the pneumothorax and the normal lung is known as the _____ _____. The lung may sometimes be identified as a _____ structure superior to the _____.

11. When _____ or _____ abdominal trauma occurs, the FAST examination may be used to locate _____ _____.

12. The examination is performed with the patient in a _____ position, but placing the patient in the _____ position shifts areas of dependency and increases the sensitivity of the FAST exam in detection of free fluid in the hepatorenal space and the perisplenic space.

13. The space located between the liver capsule and right kidney is called the _____ _____ or _____ _____.

14. When the patient is supine, the _____ is the most dependent portion of the peritoneal cavity.

15. A modified examination of the deep venous system of the lower extremities focuses on a three-point evaluation of the _____ _____ vein at the _____ junction, the proximal _____ and _____ _____ vein, and the _____ vein.

Short Answer

1. List the benefits of the FAST and eFAST examinations.

2. The presence of electrical activity without a palpable pulse being present can occur due to a number of low-flow states. List four low-flow states that can cause these findings.

3. Describe the two techniques used to evaluate for a pneumothorax with sonography.

4. List the potential spaces evaluated with a FAST examination.

IMAGE EVALUATION/PATHOLOGY

Review the images and answer the following questions.

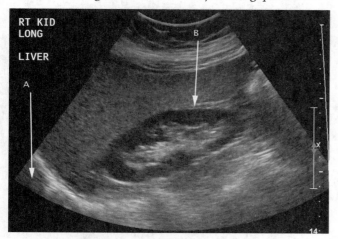

1. Name the potential space labeled *A* and the potential space labeled *B*.

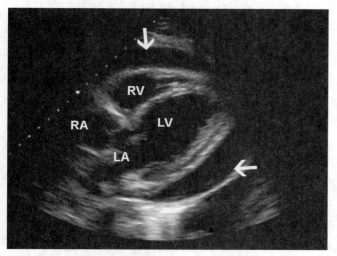

2. What are the *arrows* pointing to in this image? What condition may this lead to?

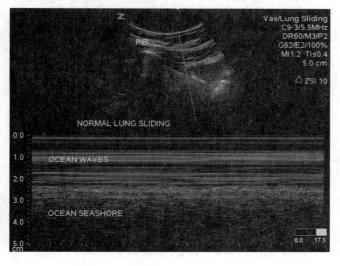

3. Describe what is seen in this M-mode image. Is this normal? How would this change if a pneumothorax was present?

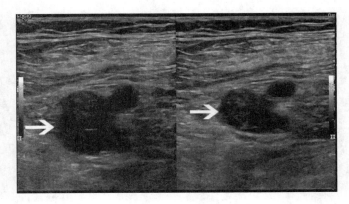

4. Describe what is seen in this split screen image of the femoral artery and vein. What technique is used here to evaluate for deep venous thrombosis?

CASE STUDY

Review the image and answer the following question.

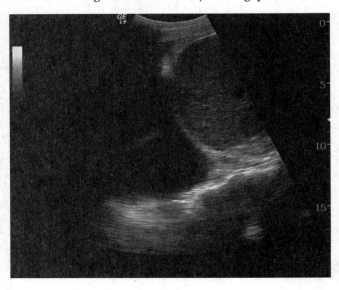

1. A patient presents to the emergency room following a severe motor vehicle accident with chest trauma from the steering wheel. This image was taken from the right upper quadrant. Describe what is seen in this image.

Foreign Bodies

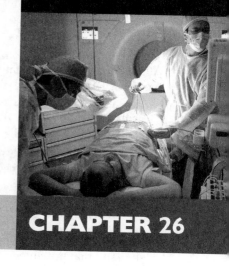

REVIEW OF GLOSSARY TERMS

Matching

Match the terms with their definitions.

KEY TERMS

1. _____ granuloma

2. _____ hyperemia

3. _____ in vivo

4. _____ in vitro

5. _____ occult

6. _____ radiolucent

7. _____ radiopaque

DEFINITION

a. Something hidden from view

b. Occurs or is made to occur within a living organism or natural setting

c. Tissue, contrast, or material that attenuates or blocks radiation; appears bright on radiograph

d. Tumor-like mass formation which usually contains macrophages and fibroblasts that form because of chronic inflammation and isolation of the infected area

e. Tissue or material that allows the transmission of X-rays and appears dark on a radiograph

f. Made to occur in a laboratory vessel or in a controlled experimental environment but does not occur within a living organism or natural setting

g. Increase in the quantity of blood flow to a body part; typically due to an inflammatory response

CHAPTER REVIEW

Multiple Choice

Complete each question by circling the best answer.

1. Which of the following materials is most likely to visualize on a radiography examination?

    a. gravel

    b. wood splinter

    c. cactus spine

    d. plastic sliver

2. Foreign bodies smaller than what size can be more difficult to detect on a sonography examination?

    a. 1 cm

    b. 7 mm

    c. 5 mm

    d. 2.5 mm

3. Which of the following statements regarding foreign bodies is FALSE?

a. Metallic foreign bodies can be easily seen with both sonography and radiography.

b. Most glass foreign bodies can be easily seen with both sonography and radiography.

c. Organic foreign bodies are the easiest to locate with radiography.

d. Inorganic foreign bodies present little challenge for sonography.

4. A patient presents with a red, painful area on the right hand that presented after working in the yard. In what phase would a foreign body be characterized if the sonogram shows a. 1.5-cm echogenic linear structure directly under the area of concern with a hypoechoic halo seen surrounding the echogenic structure, and posterior shadowing?

a. acute

b. intermediate

c. chronic

d. granulomatous

5. A patient presents with a painful area on the bottom of her foot that initially presented more than a week ago. In what phase would a foreign body be characterized if there is a palpable lump present in the area and the sonogram shows a very echogenic linear structure with a clean shadow?

a. acute

b. subacute

c. intermediate

d. chronic

6. What is the most common complication of untreated or retained foreign bodies?

a. nerve injury

b. infection

c. tendon injury

d. allergic reaction

7. Which of the following can cause false-positive findings?

a. calcifications

b. scar tissue

c. air trapped in the soft tissue

d. all of the above may cause a false positive finding

8. Which of the following is an organic foreign body?

a. bee stinger

b. glass shard

c. graphite

d. gravel

9. Which of the following does NOT describe the typical sonographic appearance of a foreign body?

a. echogenic with clean shadowing

b. hypoechoic with an echogenic ring surrounding it

c. echogenic with a hypoechoic ring surrounding it

d. echogenic with comet tail artifact

Fill-in-the-Blank

1. Whether or not a foreign body is demonstrated on a radiograph depends on the _____ of the object.

2. Radiography detects 98% of radiopaque objects such as _____, most _____, and _____.

3. A high-frequency _____ array transducer is typically used to evaluate for the presence of foreign bodies.

4. Artifacts such as _____ and _____ can be helpful in both identifying and locating a foreign body.

5. Color Doppler may be used to demonstrate _____ _____ surrounding the foreign body.

6. A radiograph can provide information regarding the _____, _____, and _____ of the foreign body. Radiographs obtained in two perpendicular projections can be used to _____ the location.

7. A foreign body will only be radiographically visualized if its density is _____ than the surrounding soft tissue.

8. When evaluating a foreign body with sonography, visualizing the foreign body _____ to the transducer is important.

9. Foreign bodies are described in one of three categories _____, _____, or _____.

10. In the intermediate phase, the air that is present in the acute phase is slowly replaced with _____; therefore, the _____ artifact is typically not present. A more pronounced _____ is seen to surround the foreign body.

11. In the chronic stage, a dense, _____ material encapsulates the foreign body. The inflammatory response can result in a clean _____.

12. Metallic and glass foreign bodies may present with _____ artifacts.

13. Using sonographic guidance for foreign body removal can result in reducing the size of the _____ with a less traumatic _____ to find and remove the material.

14. The greatest advantage of CT over conventional radiography or sonography is its capability of demonstrating foreign bodies in _____. CT can detect _____, _____, _____, and _____ in bone and muscle.

15. MRI should not be used for _____ foreign bodies.

Short Answer

1. List three types of foreign bodies radiography is likely to detect and three types of foreign bodies radiography is unlikely to detect.

2. Describe the techniques used to increase visualization of foreign bodies with sonography.

3. Describe the appearance of a foreign body in the acute phase.

IMAGE EVALUATION/PATHOLOGY

Review the images and answer the following questions.

1. What artifact is seen in this image that helps the sonographer locate the foreign body? What causes this artifact?

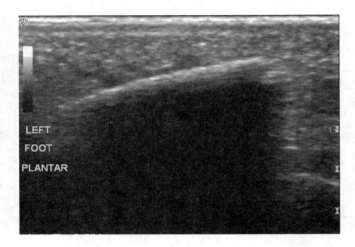

2. Describe what is seen in this image. What are the arrows pointing to? What does this represent?

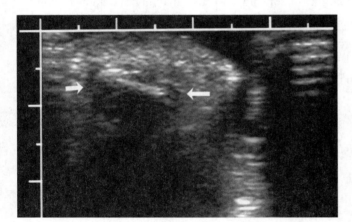

Sonography-Guided Interventional Procedures

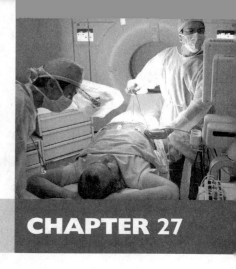

CHAPTER 27

REVIEW OF GLOSSARY TERMS

Matching

Match the terms with their definitions.

KEY TERMS

1. _____ coagulopathy

2. _____ core biopsy

3. _____ fine-needle aspiration

4. _____ fresh frozen plasma

5. _____ international normalized ratio

6. _____ partial thromboplastin time

7. _____ pneumothorax

8. _____ prostate-specific antigen

9. _____ prothrombin time

10. _____ pseudoaneurysm

DEFINITION

a. Value used to standardize prothrombin time results between institutions

b. Collection of air or gas in the pleural cavity between the lung and chest wall that creates pressure on the lung

c. Complication that can occur after cardiac catheterization or angioplasty in which a hematoma is formed by a leakage of blood from a small hole in the femoral artery

d. A defect in the body's mechanism for blood clotting

e. Lab value that can indicated the presence of prostate conditions such as prostate cancer, BPH, and prostatitis

f. PT; lab test used to evaluate for blood clotting abnormalities; the time it takes the blood to clot after thromboplastin and calcium are added to the sample

g. Procedure that uses a hollow core biopsy needle to remove a sample of tissue

h. PTT; laboratory test used to evaluate for blood clotting abnormalities

i. A form of blood plasma that contains all of the clotting factors except platelets that is used to treat patients with a coagulopathy prior to interventional procedures

j. A procedure that uses a small needle attached to a syringe; a vacuum is created and sample cells are aspirated for evaluation

CHAPTER REVIEW

Multiple Choice

Complete each question by circling the best answer.

1. Which of the following is NOT a contraindication to needle biopsy?
   a. uncooperative patient
   b. lesion deeper than 5 cm
   c. uncorrectable coagulopathy
   d. unsafe biopsy route

2. Which of the following is NOT included in a coagulation study?
   a. PT
   b. INR
   c. WBC
   d. PTT

3. Which test standardizes the results of the other coagulation studies as it adjusts for variations in processing and is expressed as a number?
   a. PT
   b. INR
   c. WBC
   d. PTT

4. Which of the following CANNOT cause a coagulopathy?
   a. blood thinners
   b. aspirin use
   c. certain antibiotics
   d. vitamin K

5. Which of the following is a procedure that uses a 20- to 27-gauge needle attached to a syringe to obtain a sample of cells for cytologic examination?
   a. core biopsy
   b. nephrostomy
   c. fine-needle aspiration
   d. paracentesis

6. Which of the following needle gauges will produce the largest specimen size?
   a. 14 gauge
   b. 16 gauge
   c. 22 gauge
   d. 27 gauge

7. Which of the following statements regarding needle visualization is FALSE?
   a. Larger caliber needles are more readily visualized than smaller caliber needles.
   b. The needle may appear as a dot or line depending on the imaging plane.
   c. The needle and transducer should be in the same plane to produce the best visualization.
   d. The more parallel the needle is to the transducer, the easier it is to visualize.

8. What is the purpose of the time-out during a procedure?
   a. Give the physician and staff a break during long procedures.
   b. Verify the correct patient is present and confirm the procedure and procedure site.
   c. Verify that all of the materials are in place for the procedure and everyone is ready to begin.
   d. Verify that the physician and staff are adequately trained in performing the procedure.

9. Which of the following is NOT one of the most common complications to occur following a biopsy?
   a. infection
   b. pain
   c. vasovagal reaction
   d. hematoma

10. Which of the following procedures is performed to remove an accumulation of serous fluid in the peritoneal cavity?
    a. thoracentesis
    b. abscess drainage
    c. nephrostomy
    d. paracentesis

Fill-in-the-Blank

1. Sonographic guidance allows for real-time visualization of the _____ _____ as it passes through tissue planes to the target area.

2. Color Doppler is used to prevent complications by identifying and helping the clinician to avoid _____ _____ that may be in the needle path.

3. A biopsy can help distinguish between _____ or _____ lesions and _____ disease.

4. Three tests _____ _____, _____ _____ _____, and _____ _____ _____ _____ measure the time it takes for blood to form a clot.

5. Patients with a coagulopathy may be given _____ _____ _____ or vitamin _____ prior to the procedure if the need for the procedure outweighs the risk of bleeding.

6. When planning a biopsy route, major _____, _____, the _____, and other _____ _____ must be avoided.

7. A _____ _____ _____ is a procedure that involves removing small samples of tissue using an automated hollow core needle commonly referred to as a _____ _____.

8. The larger samples obtained from a core biopsy are sent for a more definitive _____ evaluation. This type of procedure is commonly performed in the _____, _____, _____, _____ _____, and _____ organs.

9. The sonographic appearance of a needle is either a hyperechoic _____ or _____, depending on which imaging plane is used.

10. The sonographer's role is to recommend the _____ and _____ approach to the lesion.

11. Written _____ _____ must be obtained from the patient and everyone in the room must pause for a _____ prior to the start of the procedure.

12. Measuring the distance from the _____ to the _____ _____ will help determine the length of the procedure needle needed.

13. A needle guide that is fixed to the transducer keeps the needle _____ _____ of the transducer; however it also reduces operator freedom in choosing the _____ _____.

14. A procedure that is performed without a needle guide is considered _____.

15. A paracentesis can be performed for _____ or _____ reasons.

16. The most common causes of ascites are _____ and _____.

17. A procedure performed to remove fluid from the pleural space is called a _____. Patients are typically positioned _____, leaning over a table.

18. Indications for a prostate biopsy include elevated _____ _____ _____, abnormal _____ _____ _____, or palpable nodules. The patient is placed in the _____ _____ _____ position.

19. Percutaneous _____ injection can be used to treat pseudoaneurysms. Complications include _____ migration of the thrombin.

20. Fine-needle aspiration of thyroid nodules less than _____ is discouraged because microcarcinomas infrequently metastasize.

Short Answer

1. Describe the advantages of sonography-guided procedures over CT-guided procedures or open surgery.

2. Although sonography-guided biopsy can be used for many lesions, certain lesions may not be amenable to sonographic guidance. List three instances in which sonography-guided biopsy would not be used.

3. Discuss the reasons a biopsy of a lesion is performed.

4. List the possible complications of sonography-guided procedures.

IMAGE EVALUATION/PATHOLOGY

Review the images and answer the following questions.

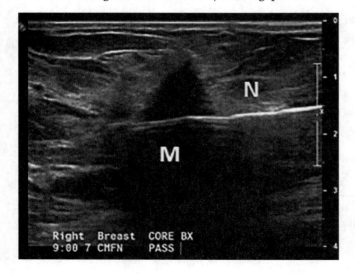

1. Is this needle (*N*) visualized in plane or out of plane? Is the needle parallel or perpendicular to the ultrasound beam?

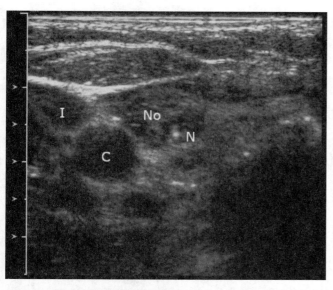

2. Is this needle (*N*) visualized in plane or out of plane? Which is easier to visualize, a needle in plane or out of plane?

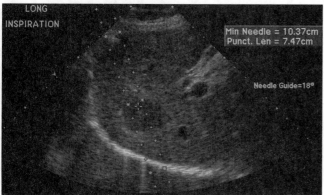

3. What do the two parallel lines represent in this image? What are the advantages of using this guide? What does the cursor between those lines represent?

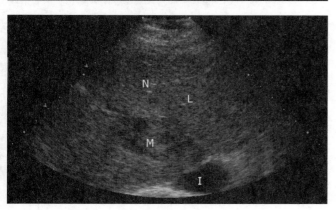

4. This image was taken in a patient undergoing a core biopsy of a liver lesion. What are the possible complications from a core liver biopsy?

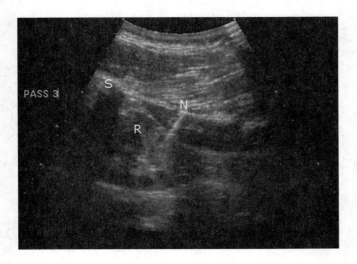

5. This image was taken in a patient undergoing a core biopsy of the kidney. List the main reasons why a biopsy of the kidney is performed. From which part of the kidney is the biopsy sample typically obtained?

CASE STUDY

Review the image and answer the following question.

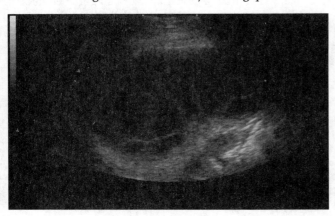

1. A patient presents with a unilateral, loculated fluid collection in the left pleural space. What are the diagnostic indications for thoracentesis? What are the complications?